LITTLE GIRL LOST

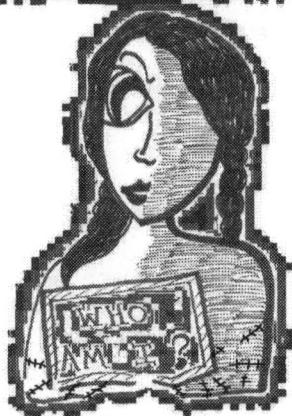

WHO AM I?

BY LOVISA PAHLSON-MOLLER

By Lovisa Pahlson-Moller

Published by:
Chipmukapublishing
PO Box 6872
Brentwood
Essex
CM13 1ZT
United Kingdom

Copyright © 2006 Lovisa Pahlson-Moller

ISBN 13:   **978-1-905610-983 2nd edition**

DEDICATION

This book is dedicated to the people I have known and loved, who have suffered with an addiction or a mental illness, and in particular to all those whose lives have ended before having a chance to see or read this book. Their lives and memories are echoed through some of these pages and poems. They will not be forgotten.

To protect the identities of certain treatment centres, hospitals etc...names and descriptions have been slightly altered. Certain names have also been changed for personal reasons or to protect identities of patients, doctors and staff.

ACKNOWLEDGEMENTS

Thank you to my beloved Rhodesian Ridgeback, Kimbo, who died on the 12th of November 2005 at 10:30pm of gastric torsion. For almost twelve years he was my best friend and the greatest companion. Without him I would have never met my boyfriend, nor would I have recovered so well from borderline personality disorder. He is loved by so many and has touched many hearts and many lives. There is a hole in the world now that he has gone. He is loved beyond understanding and apart from the odd squirrel, is missed profoundly.

Thank you to Esther Heskith for understanding me, yet never judging. I pray that your children will never walk the path that we did. Our worlds are different in some ways but their boundaries link up. My time spent in certain treatment centres would not have been the same with out you. With you I could laugh at things that would have otherwise broken me.

I'd like to give big sloppy kisses to my Westonbirt friends, Lucy Collinson, Hattie Fisher, Alice Lycette-Green and Frankie Somerset. You have all seen me change dramatically (emotionally, physically and through my image) in all the years you have known me. You have all in your own individual little ways helped me with kindness; friendship and understanding grow into a happy woman who is somewhat normal. You have all given me great memories in the past and hopefully more to come. Thanks girls for being there when I needed you and for putting up with me when I was a bitch. I love you all!

I'd like to give a big hug to Tel. Pappa Smurf. He was a man who used to live rough on the streets of London and who I got to know very well and even lived with for some time. He is a good friend, and a great listener. Apart from his sherry he loves nothing more than watching dogs play in the park. You prefer to live life, not read about it so I guess that you will never get round to reading this book, but I know that the fact that you are mentioned in it will make you happy. You always make me laugh with your silly little jokes and your unique views on life. You have a good heart and a cheerful attitude to everything that is catching. I'm glad you're off the streets. To me you are like an eccentric uncle and life is quieter, but also emptier when you are not around. Thank you for being simply...you.

I'd like to give a huge hug to D.J. Arriaga, a 24-hour nurse, my lovely shadow in Arizona. He was a staff member who really cared, not just for me, but hundreds of kids like me. Thank you so much for listening to me ramble on about everything and nothing for hours on end and still have a smile on your face. For making me laugh, and for occasionally joining in with my rebellious nature just for the fun of it. I will never forget you.

A thank you to Wendy Lader, and Caren Konterio, who run the S.A.F.E

Alternatives Program for self-harmers in Chicago. You gave me so much insight into self-harm and who I am. You helped me realise that I am not alone in my thoughts and behaviours. You showed me that there is humour in recovery, and that we can all choose which path to take in life.

To Janna Spark in London, without you this book would not have been possible. In many ways this book is like your baby as well as mine. Thank you for just being able to cope with me and for not just being a psychologist but also a good friend. For helping me grow with music when I was younger, and for making me laugh, laugh and laugh some more in sessions that were not funny, eleven years later. You had a belief in me when I doubted myself. You helped me remember that there were moments of happiness in my childhood. Thank you for not supplying me with medication, but possibly the best cookies in London.

6

I'd like to say a huge thank you to Dr. Mike McPhillips, (Doc) in London, for never sectioning me, even at my maddest moments. For helping me become aware of and understand my Borderline Personality Disorder. I have yet to come across another psychiatrist who has as much insight and ways to deal with a bpd patient as you. You always had great patience, when I was exhausting and demanding. You never gave up on me when so many other people had. Thank you for making me laugh hysterically even though not always intentionally and for helping me realise, contrary to what I once thought, that some psychiatrists are human after all, and that some can be trusted.

I'd like to say a big thank you to Françoise Von-Hurter, a good family friend who has given me great insight into the whole book world. You have given me valuable advice on the progress of my book, the legal side of things as well as putting forward many helpful ideas. Thank you for taking time to help me get published and being so supportive and understanding of what I have been through.

Thank you to Jason Pegler and Chipmunkapublishing, for letting my story and voice be heard. You are crusaders in a world that has so much judgement and your determination to tear down the stigma surrounding mental illness is inspirational.

To my darling boyfriend Marc Hamilton, my Troll, thank you for loving me, to your star and back. For being there for me when I need you the most and hugging me for hours when I'm feeling down. For making me laugh till I have tears in my eyes and I'm rolling around on the floor. For singing; you are my sunshine…my only sunshine, to me just to make me smile, for never judging me, my life, or my past. You are the most amazing, gentle and caring man I have ever known and although we have had ups and downs we always work them through. You have taught me that I am worth something and you know me better than anyone else.

You are my everything. You make me whole. You are my rock, and without you I am lost.

To my family, I thank them for supporting me and loving me. And most importantly for patiently trying to understand a world they cannot.

To my dad I want to apologise to him for any of his expectations that I could not, and perhaps will never meet. I know now that you are proud of me. When I first knew I was going to publish my diary I wanted to hurt you. I wanted to write about all the pain I felt you put me through so that you could understand how much you had hurt me in my life. Not only is that immature but also unfair. I am so happy that we are getting on better. We are both very stubborn and great at putting our views across, and in a lot of ways I am probably more like you than anyone else in the family. I do not want to hurt you. I am proud of you and sometimes I even think you are quite cool! And although I am sure we will have several more disagreements in life I am honoured to call you my dad.

I want to thank my big brother Ivan. For putting up with me when I was embarrassing, impossible and lost. Thank you for treating me like your sister and not like some nut case. I want to thank you for never failing to cheer me up with your fantastically good Rik Mayall and Blackadder impersonations and your famous woozies that never fail to leave me laughing hysterically.

I'd like to give a big hug to my little sister Kat. Twinkle toes. The last couple of years we have drifted apart when we once where inseparable and I can't help but think that if I didn't have my disorder, we still would be. Thank you for putting up with me when I was being weird and difficult. You asked me once when you had just gotten your car, Peetree, why I couldn't just be happy for you. I am, more than you will ever know. You are an amazing, bright young women and it was you who taught me that you can enjoy life no matter who or what you are. I feel so proud to call you my sister. You are, always have been, and always will be the shining star in my life.

I'd like to say a special thank you to my mom, who has supported me with endless love and compassion, and encourages me all the way in whatever I choose to do. For putting me to bed when I was like a zombie due to medication and for being able to joke about my self-harm, hallucinations and voices. Thank you for accepting that this is who I am and for believing in me and never giving up. It was your strength that gave me the will to carry on living every time I wanted to end my suffering. I love you so much and am so lucky to have you as my mum.

Foreword:

'Little Girl Lost' is an amazingly brave tale written from the heart. At the tender age of twenty two Lovisa Pahlson-Moller has experienced more than many people experience in a life time and managed to face her own fears, face up to them and begin to conquer the huge challenges that would knock the stuffing out of anyone. 'Little Girl Lost' is interspersed between wonderful articulate and heart felt prose and beautiful poems that can make the reader cry. Lovisa spent two years in several different psychiatric wards and treatment centre and managed to maintain her dignity, wit and sense of humour during these horrific times. She was diagnosed with Borderline Personality Disorder at the age of seventeen and kept a diary during her stay in boot camps, psychiatric wards and different clinics. 'Little Girl Lost' is a tear jerking roller coaster of a read which deals with the authors own tragic experiences of rape, BDP, self harm and coming to terms with being labelled with Borderline Personality Disorder. With the publication of this book Lovisa Pahlson-Moller arrives as an ambassador for other people who have experienced self harm, Borderline Personality Disorder and rape. To be able to do this at only 20 years of age in such an open, articulate and moving way is nothing short of remarkable. I expect her bravery to go on to help other people who have expereinced similar pain.

Jason Pegler CEO of Chipmunkapublishing

PROLOGUE

When I started writing this book I was overwhelmed, not just in putting it all together, but having to force myself to remember some unpleasant memories. The fact that my thoughts, experiences and inner torments would be put in black and white on paper seemed impossible at first. I was sure that I would disappoint myself and those around me, or even worse, fail.

My darkest secrets, my hidden life would be on display for anyone to read, and I was petrified of what people would think of me, my disorder, where I have been, and my world.

A big part of me wanted to reveal the true me. However I found a small part of me wanting to sugar coat everything - to down play some passages, and lie about others. I was craving to reach out to explain my life, yet I wanted acceptance.

I soon realised that if I was going to write this book, I had to be completely open and honest. If I wanted people to know, I had to be true to myself. If I desperately wanted to help myself, I had to go through the pain. There were moments when I could not bring myself to write some memories. I didn't think people would understand a mind like mine but I had to put these concerns aside. I needed to do this for me. It was hard, sometimes unbearable.

However as I became organised, determined and sure that this was what I wanted to do, I found myself becoming less worried of what people thought. I reminded myself that this book had a dual purpose: to enlighten others about some people's awful realities and to sort out the chaos of my own.

I found myself getting better. It was slow at first, but I noticed it. I still had my moods, my self- harm, my voices, but they were not as extreme. That's when I knew that this book was a way forward, my therapy.

13

That by having to remember memories that left me screaming, I had to accept them and deal with them. I could no longer block them out. There are still, and always will be experiences that I cannot, and maybe never will want to recall. There are some which are too hard for me even now to accept, let alone write down but in time I hope they do not matter.

It was only when I was getting near to the end of converting my journal into a book that a recurrent nightmare started, a weird dream. Unpleasant; the finished manuscript is on the bedside table and a horrid looking midget steals it. He starts printing out copies and sends it to thousands of people. I wake up and go to the door, only to find several crowds of people shouting at me, each with a copy in hand. Before I can do or say anything I get the finished copies thrown at me. I get battered with them, while the midget looks on, laughing.

I have learnt more things than I had hoped in doing this project. I have learnt more about myself and have come to better understand those like me. I am writing this for those who are lost, alone and feeling as desperate as I had felt.

When I was in one particular psychiatric unit I came across a book. I could relate to every page. I felt less alone. I knew that there were others like me. Hiding in locked rooms, under long sleeves, behind anything that could damage them, and I smiled knowing that I shared my world with others. I hope this book does the same to those who are living or have lived in that dark place; then not only will I have at least succeeded at my writing but also in giving them hope.

INTRODUCTION

Well, I guess you could say I didn't have a great start in life. I wasn't wanted, even as an amoeba. My birth mother had no personal drug history, or alcohol history. My blood father also didn't drink or use drugs, but was not ready for a baby. I certainly was not an immaculate conception. My birth mother couldn't handle having a child, being a mother at age 16. I understand that. She was a baby having a baby. So I got a new mother and father. However for most my childhood I didn't think of him as a father. He was there on weekends and late at night, but that was all. I have pictures of all my birthday parties. He is not in any one of them. I have pictures from school plays and ballet classes; again he is not seen in them. My most favourable memories from childhood do not include him. I didn't know him. He was the authority figure who screamed at me at bedtime when he had received my school reports. He was the man who pushed me into activities that his friend's children did. He could not understand that I was different. He thought that all my behaviour was due to lack of discipline.

It wasn't until my late teens that he finally realised that for most of my life I had had a mental disorder. He wanted to control every aspect of my life that resulted in me rebelling. Now that I am older I am on better terms with him. We laugh and joke. We talk openly about the past and we both try. We even get on most of the time and I am closer to him now through doing this book than I ever was before. However old hurts like scabs leave scars.

It wasn't until my third treatment centre that I realised I had a mental disorder. It is called Borderline Personality Disorder. It is more common in women. One doctor has said I will suffer from it for the rest of my life another has said I will have it until I am at least forty years old. Doctors never say the same thing and that makes everything confusing. I used to have it to an extreme. Several doctors told me I was one of the worst cases they had ever seen. At the time I took that as a compliment. I was always trying to get their attention by being the most demanding patient, and most often I was. I didn't understand what it was at the time. I do now after reading countless books on the subject. It was very hard to accept at first but after a while, it was a relief to know there was an explanation to why I felt the way I did and why I behaved a certain way.

So many doctors don't know how to deal with a BPD patient and I have met so many who have no idea what it is. I think this was the main factor in why I was shifted from hospital to hospital for over a year.

I was so relieved. I could finally give a name to my behaviour, my thoughts, my cutting and the voices inside my head. It gave a lot of explanation to certain childhood behaviours and why my mother had always said I was different from the other kids she had raised. Living with a severe mental disorder is hard to say the least. Some people are scared of you when they find out that you have it, others think that you are nuts and live in La La land. I do but not all the time, and that is very hard for people to understand.

If I had cancer I would be accepted. It is something everyone has heard of. They can see all the physical symptoms and hear from doctors who specialise in the field. But with a mental illness you can't see what is happening in the brain. It is not talked about, and doctors have conflicting ideas of what is best for the patient. I have learnt to accept my disorder, and to accept who I am; who I always will be and to deal with it.

So, theoretically, I hit the lottery by being adopted, by having a good mother who kept in contact with my birth mother for a while so, I haven't the unresolved mysteries of being adopted like some kids have. I became part of a family; complete with brother and three years later another adopted sister. I felt that my brother was always favoured by my father, my sister favoured by my mother. Is it any wonder that I got lost?

Maybe that lost look is something that could be seen in my young eyes, and was taken advantage by me being raped. Maybe that rape triggered the voices. Maybe the rape that triggered the voices triggered the cutting that triggered another rape years later.

I know all these maybes are true but it is beyond some people's understanding, especially my parents. In their hearts I don't think they could admit to themselves that all these things that went on in my life could have happened to their child, to their family, without them knowing about it. Because by admitting it would mean that they were bad parents. And that they would carry the blame. I don't blame them.

I did, but do not now. I believe that even if I had had the perfect parents, I would have still turned out this way. I would still have hated school and I would still have fallen in love with self-harm. *Self-harming is what I am good at. I am an expert in the art of cutting and missing veins and arteries. It is a subject that most people feel uncomfortable talking about. ....But to help children and adults suffering with self-harm, it needs to be discussed.* For me self-harming is a way of expressing my feelings. When you are depressed. When you are filled with hate, anger, rage, sorrow and sadness, it is a relief to cut or burn. To see blood is a way of releasing all emotions. A bulimic purges, an alcoholic drinks. It is a coping method that is hard to undo. Yes there are those that do it for attention, but I was never one of those people.

I hid it for many many years before confessing to my mother in a car on the way to school one morning. I was fourteen at the time and had been self-harming since the age of six. It started with pulling some milk teeth out with a hair clip. I then started scratching at my skin with a compass and scissors. When I was about

17

eleven I started cutting to release blood. I only did it about once a month. That was all I needed at the time. I would use sanitary towels to cover the small one-inch cuts. They fit snugly under my school shirt. I could then dispose of them without any suspicion from anyone. I never wanted stitches, and never really needed them until I was about sixteen. I soon realised that without stitches the scars healed badly. They were red and puffy and wide. I liked the fact that they looked so big. When you get stitches they heal into a thin white line. By the time I was eighteen and out of my last treatment centre, I was self-harming almost everyday.

I was visiting hospital emergency rooms and doctors almost weekly for bandages, tetanus shots and stitches. I often had to go to different ones in case they started wanting to section me under the mental health act of being a risk to myself. I would take my junkie friends along for support, as in the beginning I was too scared to go alone. I got bandaged up and they got clean needles. It was a good deal. I got bad mouthed by a lot of nurses and I understood why. They spent all day helping people whose lives were sometimes ruined by an accident and then I came in using up their time for something I voluntarily did. I could understand their anger but they didn't understand me and that I wasn't doing this for fun. I wasn't in control. I have even had one doctor at a hospital refuse to give me stitches and instead send me away, bleeding quite badly.

I felt ashamed of my scars, and still sometimes do, even though I shouldn't. Several scars on various parts of my body will stay with me for the rest of my life. Others will fade and disappear, leaving just a distant memory. But I strongly believe that it is not something that should be kept a secret, only to be discussed behind closed doors. Self-harmers hate talking. They feel that they cannot possibly put in words what they are going through. They need a physical way of showing their pain... To prove that they are alive and real... To show that they are not hollow inside... To numb them out and to swallow them in a state of calm...but many people don't know the shame and guilt that they feel afterwards.

So there was no point turning to my parents. They didn't understand my world. As for turning to teachers: I left school at 16, with bad exam results and due to learning difficulties I had a poor education. Some teachers even made fun of my bad spelling, and because I couldn't grasp sometimes the easiest concepts being taught in class. I did however in my school life have some very good teachers but for the most part I hated it. Some of my worst memories in life were being at school. Then again I also believe that most pupils teach the teachers. Instead I turned to people my parents would have liked to have kept me away from. Kids addicted to drugs, prostitutes and men living on the streets. I felt that they were the only ones who understood me, they accepted me more than other people did, and much to my mother's confusion, I could relate to them. My closest friend at the time was a girl called Esther who was addicted to heroin and had been to two individual treatment centres with me. I preferred to be with her than other self-harmers.

I was constantly surrounded by hard-core heroin users for about three years and never once tried it. Some of them would play tricks for cash. However I believe that if I wasn't self-harming at the time I would now be a smack head. I used to think having friends like that was cool. I changed my mind after having been to eight funerals in 2002. Almost one every other month that year and it was incredibly painful and surreal.

My boyfriend Marc was homeless when I met him walking my dog in a London park. I didn't think at the time I was worth enough to be with a man who didn't have issues. My mother at first was horrified. At the time I was twenty and Marc was 13 years older than me, and an alcoholic. He used to do crack and liked his weed. He had no family and had two children he never saw. He was involved in a court case where he was being charged with assaulting a policeman. He didn't have the best childhood and had very little faith in himself and other people. He has seen me grow each day and get stronger in my recovery. He has met people I have been in treatment centres with and saw Esther's daughter get christened. He has encouraged me and pushed me towards happiness. Light can come out of darkness and he has been a huge influence in me getting better from my disorder. Although an alcoholic and a crazy girl isn't a children's fairytale story, I did get my happy ever after.

I have come a long way to realise that dare I say it, yes I dare: I'm normal. I'm not insane. I'm not normal. I am insane. Okay so I go back and forth.

Maybe I vacillate because I think my confidence level is pretty shaky, at times low, but there are other times that for the first time in my life, in 22 years that I am actually happy. For the first time I have found a man who understands me, who I love. He is a man who I can talk to without fearing judgement or abuse. He loves me for who I am.

I know now that there are many worlds in this one world, and I dwell in many. I also know that that is true for many people and not just me. However I also know that not many people have the insight that I have. I feel I have the same knowledge at age 22, that most people don't get until they are a lot older. I have lived so many lives in my short time. I was grown up, before hitting puberty. At an age when boys, dates, and going to clubs should be on my mind, I want to settle down and start a family. I have lived already. I was doing those things years ago. Most my friends are not younger than 30 years old. These are the people I can relate to. I am a wise old woman stuck in this young girl's body. So in some ways, this hell that I have been through, this life that I have led has provided me with a perspective that very few people have. I used to think I was damned. But now, am I blessed?

In my time in treatment centres, hospitals, psychiatric wards and rehabs I have been on lots of medication. Some helped and others didn't. I have been on things like Seroxat/Paroxotine, and Promazine/Sparine that made me worse than I already was. My urge for self-harming became greater and my voices louder. Then there was Risperidone/Risperdal that calmed my voices and slowed my racing thoughts into slow motion. Then there was Prozac/Fluoxetine, which did nothing at all. Trazodone/Molipaxin had a side affect that helped me sleep. I was at one point on the highest dose a nurse had ever issued. I was once given an alcoholic's Temazepam for two weeks by mistake before my doctor realised. Zopiclone/Zimovane was also given to me at one point to help me sleep, which worked but it gave me a horrible metal taste at the back of my mouth that intensified when I had a cigarette. There was Seroquel/Quetiapine, which I loved but after being on it for a while made me lactate! And then towards the end of my recovery I was on things like Cipramil/Citalopram and Olanzapine/Zyprexa that at one point I could have happily married, they helped so much but it gave me an incredibly low sex drive. I was on other things that I cannot remember now.

Some were given to me as a one off, when I was getting violent or just very stressed out. Others where tried and quickly switched for another type. I have had nurses tell me that I shouldn't worry about what I was taking and have been refused the names of some. The reasons why I do not know.

My view on medication is that in a lot of cases it helps and people who go around advertising that no patient should be on it is dangerous. There are pills out there that can distort the mind and make you worse than you were to start with. Given to those who are too young or not suited...but then there are some which have saved me from doing stupid things that could have ended my life. I think it varies from person to person and that you have to hope that your psychiatrist or doctor knows what he or she is doing. Esther was once given the wrong meds and was crawling around on all fours like a dog for hours before almost drowning in a bath tub on a hospital ward. Another man I know came into the ward for depression and after having been given a very high dose of a junkies detox medication fell down and broke his leg badly. The nurses after having refused responsibility and an ambulance ordered him a black cab to the nearest hospital, leaving him having to pay for it. I have been off all medication for about two years now. Right now I do not need it. But will I in the future? Maybe.

Chapter One - My World

Ever felt sad and been so down, that to carry a smile is impossible? Has time ever stopped without a reasonable explanation? Where a few hours could have passed, or even a day, and there is no memory of how you spent that time of blackness?

Is your best friend or dearest enemy a disfigured shadow? Something your mind has created, and others cannot see or hear? Have you ever placed your life in a bottle of pills? Can you not tell the difference from a dream or reality? Do your emotions reflect from the blade of a knife? Have you ever felt sadness in others joy, or joy in your own pain? Ever not feared death, but life itself? I have…this is my life…welcome to my world…

MY FIRST SELF-HARM.

Sitting in the darkness,
Lit up by the moon,
There is a little girl,
Who grew up way too soon,

Sitting in the darkness,
Surrounded by despair,
There is a little girl,
Who keeps pulling out her hair,

Sitting in the darkness,
Glancing at her reflection,
There is a little girl,
Who craves for protection,

Sitting in the darkness,
A sharp hair clip in hand,
There is a little girl,
Who doesn't understand,

23

Sitting in the darkness,
Stabbing at her mouth,
There is a little girl,
Who pulls her teeth out,

Sitting in the darkness,
Filled with fear,
There is a little girl,
Who cannot cry a tear,

Sitting in the darkness,
Watching her own blood flow,
There is a little girl,
Who can't make her troubles go,

Sitting in the darkness,
Afraid to go to bed,
There is a little girl,
Who smiles at stains of red,

Sitting in the darkness,
Her mouth filled with pain,
There is a little girl,
Who wants to start again,

Sitting in the darkness,
Constantly banging her head,
There is a little girl,
Who wishes she were dead,

Sitting in the darkness,
Not uttering a sound,
There is a little girl,
Who will never be found.

Idaho-1 Boot Camp.

October-December
17 years old

Arrival: Frostbite on my feet, snow everywhere, and I arrive in leather platform sandals and a snakeskin printed short skirt. I am wearing a low cut revealing top and a short fluffy jacket. I look like I have been picked up off a street corner, minus the stockings. My hair is very long and multi-coloured. It looks like I am carrying a rainbow's nervous breakdown on my head. I am not a happy bunny!

25/10/00-8/9/00, 06:00am
This is the time most of us wake. Some in fear, even in tears waiting the exhausting day that lies ahead of them. We wake up from the cold. The campfire outside has burned throughout the night and has now been put out. The dry smoke enters the tepees we sleep in causing us to cough and our eyes to sting.

We hear mumbling from the drill sergeants taking hand over from the night staff. Sometimes we can make out a name, and if we recognise our own we hope it is not to be used for punishment. Those of us who have been here a while quickly and quietly sneak on our trousers inside our sleeping bags in preparation of the wake up call. A selected staff member will collect our boots that have been lying in a pile being guarded by the night staff. The point being that if we try to run away during the night in meters of snow with just socks on our feet, we will freeze and turn back.

First Impression: Not a hospital. I thought it was the army. It was very, very cold. This is not what I signed up for. I do not call this an outdoor experience. This is the modern version of a concentration camp, minus all the barbed wire. At least they are not that sadistic.

It's 06:30am. When we hear the staff yell wake up call we have just five minutes to get up, change, tie our boots, stuff the sleeping bags into their small cases, roll our bed mats, fold our duffle bags, finish our water bottles, sweep our sleeping area, tie our rain gear at our waist, and round up in circles on the decks.

If we do not do it in time we must redo it over and over until we get it right. Then we must pass inspection. The staff make sure our bottles are empty, our hair not sticking out from our hats, our boots tied correctly and that we have our chains on the bottom of our boots. They help us not slip when running on ice. Then the tepees are checked. If our areas our not plum and square we start again. If this happens it will disturb the whole day, as it is run with precision to time keeping.

Then we do check out. This means we stand in circles and scream out our group names. It was Otters for the girls and tatonkas for the boys. Then we run in single file to the water pump, our eyes on the head in front. When running, if we look elsewhere or at the boys we must do ten minutes of push-ups with our eyes closed.

Then we wash up, fill our water bottles and start the humiliating experience of using the bathroom. Here we call them potties, and have to spend no more than thirty seconds using them. If we need longer time we must scream out to the whole camp that we are doing a number two, and ask permission to spend longer, hoping we are granted this. If we are very delayed for breakfast the camp yell back no. The same goes if we have our period.

We then scrub them clean, disinfect each one and sweep the concrete surrounding them. Then we line up single file, run to the mess tent where we circle up again and do another check out.

07:00am
For breakfast we have to eat two bowls of oatmeal and a piece of fruit. We also have to finish our bottles. We drink about five a day. That's on average two to three

litres a day. We work hard and it is very cold up here so we feel sick from dehydration otherwise.

If we are caught glancing at the boys or swear, we have to take our plate outside and eat our meal in the snow. If a certain table is being too loud during breakfast they have to carry the solid wood, heavy table down the steps of the mess tent and outside. Sometimes if there are only a few people sitting at the table we have to volunteer to help. Usually it will take twelve of us to manage it.

07:30am
This is the time where we have to clear the tables and sweep the floor. Also we have to wash every plate by hand. There is not much electricity here so we have to boil the water before using it. Then we have to run to the water pump, fill our bottles and brush our teeth over a bucket.

08:00-10:30am
After breakfast we have physical workout (pt.) we do sit ups, push ups, aerobics, star jumps, running on the spot and jogging round the centre of the base camp. We have to pace ourselves but we are not allowed to stop for the entire pt session. Two months before I arrived, a boy died from a heart attack. They pushed him too hard. In fact most of the new people who first arrive are sick in the first week.

A boy almost froze to death last Christmas when he tried to escape. And a girl who tried to do a runner last summer, was chased by a bear and then mauled by a mountain lion. She however survived. They found her and she was taken to the hospital. When she had recovered they sent her back here! Then again rumours are rumours.

10:30-11:00am
This is when we get to rest for half an hour. We do stretches and slowly walk around. Then we are allowed to sit in the snow to cool off. The staff say that if we get

too hot when the air is so cold we can get ill. We drink more water and practise breathing exercises.

11:00-12:00pm
After we have cooled down we have work detail to do. This means we haul in tree trunks into the boot camp, carry and fetch buckets of water, collect our lunch in wheelbarrows, maul wood, saw logs, and clean the camp. It's such hard work and your arms are left aching. You get blisters all over your hands. Then we wash up fill our bottles and circle up by the mess tent.

The Professionals: I saw the Psychiatrist about half an hour every week. Little did I know that that was considered alot. The staff believed that discipline could change an addiction, or coping strategy. They thought that I was an alcoholic. ...and that cutting was an addiction, both psychological and biological. They couldn't figure it out themselves, even though I knew it was psychological because if I stop self harming, I won't go onto any kind of physical craving but my mind is almost magnetically attracted to it. Why didn't they know this? What did they know? They may have known several theoretical ways or strategies to deal with rebellious teenagers but I didn't think any of their approaches were right for me. They not only didn't know about self-harming, they didn't get it right about the alcohol. I wasn't an alcoholic, I almost was. But I wasn't a hundred percent.

This was the first time of many times I have been misdiagnosed and treated for the misdiagnosis. In my experience very few professionals appreciate how awful it is to be labelled. It makes you feel like an outcast. It is even worse, though, when you are labelled and they are wrong. I felt stigmatised. Unfounded labelling should be a punishable crime.

12:00-12:30pm

At this time we have lunch. We get a salad, a sandwich and a piece of fruit. If it is very cold we get to have soup instead the sandwich. We don't get desserts or seconds.

On Saturday mornings we do get pancakes and syrup in the morning because right afterwards we have a serious and very hard four and a half hour pt session which almost leaves everyone crying. In that group we have to run a mile in snow as well as other stuff like pulling a tree trunk down a dirt road. You have to do it on your own and know one has managed to pull one more than a meter.

12:30pm
After lunch we have to wash all the plates again, sweep the mess tent and brush our teeth. Usually in the afternoons it snows a lot so we all put on our rain clothes. We then shovel salt on the grounds of the camp. When it snows we can't see where the ice is, and have to put on our second pair of gloves. We then get inspected to make sure we still look tidy and neat.

We also get foot checks at every meal and at night. We have to take both our boots and socks off. A drill sergeant will press all your toes to make sure you have good circulation. If your toes don't go pink once pressed you have to do five minutes of exercises. They also check our fingers, noses, cheeks, and ears.

01:00-03:00pm
During this time we have raps. They are like therapy sessions. It is the only time we can look at the boys, and say whatever we want. We are allowed to just scream if we need to. They often all ask us about our parents and our childhood. It's fairly boring.

It is this time of the day that a restraint might happen. The staff will pin you to the ground if you are too aggressive. When you have calmed down, a small group of staff members will sit down with you and talk

29

about your issues and concerns. I only got restrained once when I beat up a female drill sergeant. They don't get angry with you though. They will often take someone out to the woods to talk so that they can just get away from camp a short while.

We also use this time to get checked by the doctor, and speak to a psychiatrist. We also get all our stuff searched. Often the guys will have hidden fruit in their duffle bags if they are planning to run away. Other people might have taken a knife if they are planning to hurt one of us, or a staff member. We also get weighed.

03:00-04:00pm
It starts to get dark at this time. We spend this hour mauling hundreds of logs so we can stay warm at night. The staff light torches so we can see our way around.

We also go and collect more food for dinner. It gets even colder and we have to close the openings to the tepees so small bugs won't fly in. We then collect out dirty laundry and give them to the staff. We collect a clean pair of underwear and head to the showers.

04:30pm
We get to have a shower every other night. The boys go one day, the girls go another. The shower house is a short trek from the camp and we run there single file to keep warm. Usually four female staff will take us depending on the group size. When we get there we hang up all our clothes and strip off naked in front of everyone. It is awkward at first but you get used to it.

We then line up so the staff can check us for any bad blisters, or foot sores, and nits. They spray our feet with disinfectant. They also take this time to cut hair. The boys get theirs shaved into a crew cut and the girls have there's cut to chin level unless their parents object. They cut all mine off. It was multi coloured when I first arrived so they dyed it a horrid brunette colour,

30

which looks more like dark green. We also get our nails cut short.

Those that self harm get checked for the progress in their wounds healing, but also to make sure they haven't done any recent ones. We also get a body search. We have to spread our legs in front of everyone while a nurse checks for weapons.

We get five minutes to shower. The boys get two, as they don't need to wash their hair. We don't get any deodorant so everyone smells. The shampoo and soap is a powder than turns to liquid when wet it gives me rashes, it's horrible.

After the shower we have to mop the floors of the room. We all have to be ready, washed and changed in half an hour.

The Other Patients: There was a cocktail of teenagers in the camp. Some were there for genuine attitude and/or behavioural problems. These would consist of being aggressive towards teachers at school, ignoring their parent's rules, putting themselves in danger through drug and alcohol use, stealing cars and frequently getting arrested. Then there were those who were put there as a sharp wake up warning, the youths who would soon end up on a downward path. They would surround themselves with negative friends and have a poor attitude about school, life and their family.

However there was the occasional teenager who was placed there for a small purpose such as failing to meet their parents expected school grades or simply being disobedient at times. These parents who could not understand how their child could not meet their expectations would simply presume that a boot camp should sort out all the problems for them. There were also a handful of kids that were placed in the camp with minor to moderate mental problems. In time they would be transferred to a suitable hospital that would be able to meet the needs of the person in ways a boot camp couldn't.

They would often then be transferred to a secure unit or hospital closer to their home where they could get the support from their families. I became friends with the group I was in but only stayed in contact with one girl. The staff called us Tweedle Dum and Tweedle Dee, from Alice in Wonderland, we were always together. She was younger than me by a few years but had a mature mind. Last I heard she was sixteen, had run away with a bloke some years older and was getting married.

05:00-05:30pm
We all round up in a circle outside the mess tent we finally have dinner and everyone is starving. Because it gets to freezing levels we get warm food usually meat, vegetables and fruit. Everyone is so tired that we don't really speak much and the staff are also more relaxed. We drink our water and then we all have to say a goal for the next day and something we learned or appreciated today.

THE VOICES

There's a burning in my heart... Distant and yet so close... A race... It beats harder. My mind is not quite clear, yet acts on automatic reflex. My hands are shaking and waiting for the deed. Eyes dazed, focusing on nothing. My conscience coming to a final decision.

"Do it!" the voices edge me on. I give in just to shut them up. Then, there was the coolness of the razor's edge. The pressure on its plastic handle. The way it slices, so smoothly. Not jagged or uneven, but parallel lines of emotions. Bright red symbols of pain. Scarlet streams, speeding down my arm. Rivers of feelings that finally see freedom, from the prison of my tortured body.

I recognise the familiar stains. I pretend to not notice their shadows in the silvery blade. Try and remind my self, they are only hallucinations. They are only in my mind. But for some thing not real, they are all too powerful. They pull me into their distorted world like a puppet. I dress my battle wounds, and secretly know. That yet again they have won.

05:30-06:00pm
After dinner we clean up as usual. We make sure the kitchen is very clean so mice and rats won't come in. We also take out the rubbish to a shed. Sometimes we see a bear sniffing them, but they usually then run and run when they see us. We also wash up and brush our teeth. If there isn't enough wood some people are picked to maul some.

The Regular Staff: Most of the staff there were strict and believed that the best way of getting their point across was by yelling and spitting in your face. However once you had been there a while and as long as you had made progress they started to respect you.

We felt that we had become better young adults and the staff showed us this by giving us small tasks of responsibility. In their eyes we could now be trusted to fully co-operate with the program and its rules, no matter how severe they seemed to an outside audience. And it was after, and only after we had reached that stage in the camp were we listened to and respected as teenagers with real emotional and behavioural problems. That was when the staff stopped being seen as authority figures and started becoming our teachers and friends. They then started to help us in the transition of dealing with our difficulties in life.

06:00-07:30pm
We take this time to receive letters from our family, and to write back. We work on assignments and journal time. We hear readings on the native Indians, and their way of life. A lot of things at boot camp are based on them. We sometimes do beadwork if our hands don't

33

hurt too much. We prepare for course and talk about plans after our time here is up. We get more foot checks and some people get medication for different reasons. We also try to unwind for the day because we are all exhausted.

07:30pm
We go to the tepees and round up in a circle. We do a quiet check in. We do the same things but whisper our group names. We discuss the high and low points of the day. Then we go into the tepees and take off our boots. All pairs are counted. Then we get into our cold sleeping bags. We sleep on wood floors that are cold as well. The staff go to do handover to the night staff. If we are caught talking we all have to get up at 05:00am.

Departure: My lovely hair gone. GONE. Simply cut off. I look like a man from the American army. No longer does a rainbow live on me. It has been evicted and replaced by a rather nasty brown, green attempt of a colour. My clothes are all gone. GONE. Thank god they were cheap anyway. I am dressed like an army man too. A warm jacket and hat. Tied laces, short tied laces. Too short to be a suicide risk. Shirt tucked in. I am the walking definition of what they call "plum and square." My sanity gone. GONE. It has left. It has flown to someone more deserving. I am no longer known as Lou but loopy Lou. I am now qualified to be nuts. I am nuts. I must be. And I am still not a happy bunny!

THE MASK I WEAR: Don't be fooled. Don't fall for my innocent smile. There is a demon hiding behind it. You know my history and the fact that I need help. You have seen my scars and heard my diagnosis. And yet you think I am sweet, and could not hurt a fly.

Surprise is the look I get when I show my darker side. It is something I have failed to ever understand. I don't warn but instead admit to the fact that I occasionally flip out. It is written down with a question mark beside it.

You think you know me and that we have built a relationship on trust. Believing you have tamed this so called violence, if it was even there at all. My every behaviour and action is apparently predictable, and if not you can look it up. You think you have heard all my secrets and know my thoughts.

Have you learned nothing in all the years you have had this job? Nothing in human nature is predictable. To listen to someone for a few minutes or hours for a month or a year, means you know them? What does your instinct say? I'm sorry; I forgot for a brief moment that you live your life with the knowledge of experience, what books say and by listening to experts.

So then let's go on fact. If it is a fact that I have hurt and damaged human flesh, then why are you so special? You are not my friend and you have not lived in my world.

Do you really think a patient like me cannot play with you and your own emotions? Do you think that when I am sitting in that chair laughing, I actually think you are funny? When I open up and ramble on about my concerns I am not playing you? That I trust you?

What makes you so sure? The fact that you have passed the exams, seen others like me, done the lectures and read the books? Do you not consider that I too can analyse, make mental notes and also predict? There are different types of patients, and different types of professionals. Those like me have a degree in treating them.

So no, I do not think you are a balanced individual. The fact that you are a woman does not mean you understand me. I do not think you are good at your job, if you were I would not be sitting here pretending to listen to you. I would be locked up again.

I am an expert at my job, and I am just using you. I never fail to surprise. You however have not yet shown that reaction. In time though I will make sure you do and it will be my greatest accomplishment.

My View on the Place: Although many people feel that a safe, disciplined and active environment would help their out of control teenagers, many don't realise just how traumatic this could be for their child. Not only do they not realise that the quick fix solution is nonexistent but I feel that it is sad that parents these days do not wish to try and resolve their teenager's behaviour themselves. In just sending them off for someone else to deal with is not solving any issues but simply creating new ones. If a parent has tried to deal with his or her teenager's attitude and behaviour. If their ways of discipline are unsuccessful, then I feel that for some, a boot camp can be helpful. I also think that it is extremely important for the parent/s to actually see the boot camp before sending any child there. The sad fact is that there are too many unlicensed instructors working or managing these camps. The amount of mental, physical and even sexual abuse that goes on in some of these camps is far too much.

How It Affected Me: I have mixed feelings on how it affected me. It certainly gave me a wake up call. It gave me discipline that I still think I didn't need. It gave me more respect for myself and I started to realise that what I had once considered to be impossible tasks, I could do. It gave me a chance to really reflect on my life, and helped me to make some important decisions about my future. I made some good friends, both staff members and other patients. I grew to notice how much my mother had supported me and how my father had not. In the beginning I hated it and I felt that I didn't need to be there. My problems were not behavioural but mental. The camp could only help me with this to a certain point. I felt proud of myself for being able to finish the program.

I have unpleasant memories from my experience that I try not to think about. One was when I threw a punch at a drill sergeant. This resulted in my first physical restraint. However it made me aware of how violent I can get if I let things get bottled up inside for too long. In whole I think it was a good experience that gave me lessons in life that I still use today.

If I had never been sent to a boot camp I would still be living without an understanding of whom I am and who a part of me will always be. I would have never have started my roller coaster ride of treatment centres, and I would still be miserable. Perhaps the most important thing that I would never have done was to write this book.

DEATH

Death awaits me,
It creeps closer and closer.
I shut my eyes, I see things,
Are they real?
My life is just a nightmare,
Faded by self-medication,
And blocked out by pain.
My future, a chapter,
Already written by doctors.
I'm just waiting to escape it,
But miracles do not find me,
And I do not find them…ever.
So it's up to me to stop my life.

DEATH IS

Death is the beginning,
Death is the end,
Death is understanding,
Death is my only friend.
Death is the answer,
Death is the way out,
Death is the cure,
Death screams and shouts.
Death is a blade,
Death is a game,

Death is a reward,
Death carries blame.

REVENGE

I sit back with this gun,
And a large bag of bullets,
I'll be in your house when,
You walk through the door,
Two shots easy then,
You'll be lying on the floor,
But that would not be justice,
For what you did to me,
I would cut up your main arteries,
And torture you slowly,
Knock you down and pour,
Acid in both your eyes,
Then cover you with gasoline,
And watch the fire rise!
I'll put you out before you die,
Then do it again,
Till you can't even cry,
Finally when you are cold and gone,
And you smell like burnt roast,
I'll kill myself,
So I can slaughter your ghost.

NOT UNDERSTANDING

People whisper behind your back,
Not noticing you heard,
They see you and just smile,
But secretly think you're absurd,
People look at you differently,
Now they've seen the cuts,
The school says it's for attention,
Your classmates think your nuts,
Teachers call up your parents,
And give them all the blame,
I get told to start behaving,
To stop playing this game,
I get taken to the nurse,

Who examines me with disgust?
But notices some scars are old,
I tell her there's no one I trust,
So now I have a label,
Stuck permanently on my back,
I say years from now I'll still have it,
My body still under attack,
Different, crazy, delusional,
That's what the doctors see,
But I'm not one in a hundred,
For there are millions like me.

HIM

I'm waiting for the time,
To ultimately challenge him,
I'm sick and tired,
Of meaningless threats,
I want to beat him into submission,
I want to fight him unto his death,
To me he is the devils face,
That's swarming through my mind,
I need to detach him,
Physically from my life,
I need to finish him,
With power and meaning,
I won't be satisfied till I
Can see and taste blood gleaming.

IN PAIN!

I'm hurting and I'm crying,
There's a pain deep inside,
When memories fill me,
There's nowhere I can hide,
I have no comfort,
Just sadness and no joy,
I go back to every time,
I get treated like a toy,
No one hears my calling,
No one hears my screaming,
I turn to my razor or knife,

The men make my blood streaming,
It's waiting to be released,
The only thing I trust,
I feel I deserve it,
And so I know I must,
Will I ever be able to stop?
Or will I one day die,
Go too deep on a vein,
Or just find another guy,
I'm hurting and I'm crying,
There's a pain deep inside,
When memories fill me,
There's nowhere I can hide.

CHAPTER TWO

Idaho-2 Mental Hospital.

December-March
17 years old

Arrival: I sat on a chair that was bolted down to the floor, not knowing what to do. I couldn't understand what I had done to be put in a place like this. I was not like these people, was I? I was not mad. I was not insane. For that is why these places exist. For those who do not know what normal is. For those who live in their own little world. But then again I do not know what normal is either. And although I act like I live in this world I do not. Everyone here is glaring at me with those drooping eyes. Some are even dribbling. The staff had to move me across to the other side of the room to stop the male patients from trying to touch me. I do not like it here. I am not one of them. I might be crazy but I am not mad.

THE JOURNEY

It looked normal enough. From the parking lot it could have passed for a large bungalow. I guess because that's what it was. It wasn't like the type you see in the movies, the kind that's a tall white building with patrolling security guards. It wasn't until you got up close to it that you saw the few barred windows and the clown faces that banged at the windows and pulled their pants down at frightened visitors.

On the way here I had searched through my stuff to try and find some pills, anything. I only found some painkillers, so I took all I had, which wasn't much. It just seemed like the thing to do. The escorts kept trying to find out why they were taking me to a nut house. They said what everyone said, "You seem normal enough." I looked in the rear view mirror, so I was eye to eye with the driver, and quoted a line I'd read somewhere, "sometimes I am not myself, I am someone darker."

41

First Impression: Heavy chains. There were heavy chains for heavy keys, heavy keys for heavy doors. Tunnels filled with heavy doors, with heavy windows displaying heavy tragic scenes. Scenes I do not want to see…. Corridors… I am in a twisted hamster cage. I can't get out. Worse than movies and horror films. This is real. This is where the mad go. This is my new home.

THE ENTRANCE

When you entered the building, and after you had walked through several corridors with different doors that needed identification to pass through, you got to the Adolescent psychiatric. You then had to pass through two locked, heavy glass doors with about a meter between them to enter the acute unit. It was made to look nice for visiting parents. Hand drawn pictures on the wall above the nursing station and a cheerful yellow carpet. On closer observation though, you could see that all the windows and doors that were made out of glass, had wire mesh running through them. The black-patched lines made the glass shatter proof and no matter how hard you tried to break them, no one had ever succeeded.

There was the nursing station with the emergency, under the counter alarm buttons that we didn't find out about until Jack managed to get behind the desk in search for something sharp, and pressed them all.

December 8th, 2000.
I feel like a zombie. I don't know if what I'm writing will make any sense. I have been here for about five days…I think. I'm not sure, there seems to be nothing with the day or date on it. When I first got here, they did the usual spread your legs strip search. I hate those! They put me on so many pills I can't even remember some of them. The one's I can are, Seroxat, Risperidone for my voices, and Trazodone to help me sleep. I also have to wear these blue clothes that they

call whites, or scrubs. They look like the type surgeon's or nurses wear. I have to wear hospital underwear too, that itches like hell. The bras don't have under-wire in them because they say I could take my eye out with them.

They have put me in the time out room until I have, "rested". What they mean is until they know I won't kill myself. I know the walls are like this so you can't hurt yourself but I hate it. It makes me feel like I'm crazy. All I have in here is a mattress, and a pillow that is covered in plastic, and a thin blanket that gives me rashes.

Right now I'm in the classroom. We have art. It is supposed to be therapeutic and you're meant to draw your feelings. However if they catch you drawing anything they consider as "bad" they rip it up. The staff says it is a way of acting out. It is such a dumb system. If you draw a stupid rainbow they think you are improving, but no one draws those. If they catch me even writing this they'll get mad, and take it away from me.

SECLUSION

There were the three rooms in the mill area that were empty except for a mattress, which was covered in plastic in case of accidents. They were washed daily by some chemical that made the rooms smell weird. The rooms had stains in them that you couldn't identify and scribbled words or sentences. Usually some one boasting about how many restraints they had been in. The staff called them time out rooms or seclusion. The patients called them the screamers or howlers. Probably because every one put in them usually yelled their lungs out. They were supposed to be sound proof. They weren't.

Most patients had a preference to which one they wanted to be in. The one closest to the nursing station was the one where Ray, a fourteen year old, who was

43

put in here for molesting and attempting to rape his three year old sister, almost spent six months at one stage. When he left, after being transferred to a maximum security ward in Boise, it became mine. I liked it the best, as it was the only one with a window and a toilet. It also had little scribbled messages behind the door that Ray and others had managed to write, and that the cleaners either couldn't get rubbed off, or left them there in memory.

December 2000.
I have finally moved into one of the bedrooms. I have a roommate called Kaela. She is 16 and is in for smack, and cutting. Strange that for being an addict and cutter she is in a nut house! The nurses won't tell me her disorder but apparently she has no emotions or conscience. They say that if she sees some one die, she won't cry and that she doesn't feel happy when she should etc...that to me seems fucked up.

Why would she be a cutter if she has no emotions? She seems to be filled with feelings. Kaela's from Chicago, and has been here for about six months. My other roommate is called Ally. She is 17, an alcoholic and takes crystal meth like I smoke cigarettes. She was put in here for fucking her dad. Apparently he was put nowhere. She lives on the Cordelain reservation. Her excuse for drinking is that she's half Indian, and she claims that if you were to slice her arms, vodka would run from her veins.

Ally has been here about a year. She spends her days on the social unit. That's were they send you if you are almost able to go home. She sleeps here though because she flips out at night. She is a complete bitch and when I'm sleeping will just thump me really hard. I have panic attacks before going to bed now. She is really nice sometimes, but then suddenly she'll just flip out at me. She has two half brothers that live with their mother in New Mexico and a half sister who lives with her grandparents in Alaska.

The head nurse says that Ally thinks I am someone else and I should remind her who I am when she does it, but that never works. Other times she will sit in a corner and cry like a four year old for hours. At other times when she thinks she is close to being discharged she will try and grab the resident psychiatrist's dick. That way he will make sure she is here for a little while longer. We all think he doesn't get any action from his wife. We overheard a nurse say that his wife is suffering from sexual anorexia. Now we all call him desperate doc.

December 2000.
I have just found out that Kaela is a major bulimic. She purges like eight times a day. Well she used to, now she is restricted from the bathroom until two hours after meals. She still manages to do it in the showers at night. Even with a one-to-one, she can do it really quietly and doesn't need her fingers. She just pulls her head forward and it comes up, it's actually fairly amazing.

Ally is still being a bitch, and I now have five purple bruises on my right leg and upper back. I'm getting really scared of her. She's really creepy. She just acts like a different person and when I confront her about it, she acts as if she doesn't know what I'm talking about. I might start cheeking my meds, although that's almost impossible. First you have to roll up your sleeves, then after taking the pills, you have to lift your tongue up, and they take a torch and check behind every tooth and down your throat. Then you have to look down and vigorously shake your head so they can see if anything will fall out or not.

We had a group today about rape. This massive ex-neo Nazi guy called big Jared took it. He is fucking huge, with a baldhead, and Celtic tattoos. He still has a white power one on his arm that he has to cover up, but shows off anyway. He is a reformed rapist and has spent loads of time in the penitentiary. He was taking the group as proof that some guys can change, as

45

some guys in here have raped, or attempted to. Big
Jared was explaining that it wasn't their fault as if they
couldn't help almost fucking girls to death. I think it's
sick. The only nut jobs in here seem to be the staff.

SECURITY

There were mirrors everywhere - along the corridors,
above the nursing station, by every door and on every
corner. They didn't do much use. They never caught
Farley coming into me and Kaela's room or catch AJ
trying to push a nurse's hairpin threw his dick. The
mirror's in our rooms weren't large and shinny like the
security ones, they were blurred and made from some
kind of thick metal. They made your face look funny like
the ones you find at a carnival. We used to joke that
they were the only mirrors in the world that actually
made an anorexic look fat.

By the nursing station was a board with our names,
age, date arrived, and disorders. The disorders section
was initials only. Like a secret language that only the
mental health technicians and nurses understood. They
didn't like to put our discharge dates on, and it was
seldom that patients were given one. You would be
there until they thought you were safe, better or you got
transferred. When you reached eighteen that's what
happened. That's what we hated. The fear of adult
psychiatric was intense among every one and you
always heard scary stories about it. The thought of old
psycho men on the same ward as me, scared me
shitless. The fact that you would be locked up with
these people was more like a nightmare than a
thought.

CHECKS

It was hard to get away with anything, because of
checks. When you first arrived you were put on 5
minutes. Then be upgraded to 15mins, then finally
30mins. Checks were annoying. They woke you up at
night. After a while you would learn to be able to do a

46

deep cut in 5mins. You would have to know exactly what you were going to do, then after five, you would set up the tools in the bathroom, and then go back to your bed. Then again they would come in. When they had left you had five minutes to do a cut, throw up, whatever. No one in here got better. We just learnt to be the best at whatever it was we did. We learnt how to do everything with out being caught.

December 2000
It's art again. I am sitting at a table with Kaela and a massive girl called Ashley. Ashley has been here about two years and is a dyke in every way, to the point where you actually wonder if she has a dick. She doesn't even think of herself as a girl, and keeps making passes at me. Most girls in here munch carpet, but me. It was funny at first, but now it is really annoying. She just doesn't take a hint. She is also a compulsive liar. Nothing small, I mean everything she says is a lie, and she will defend it with her life if you act as though you don't believe her. Ashley is very intimidating but if she doesn't stop trying to feel me up I'm going to stab her, I swear.

I'm sitting next to a Tec called Matt, although we all call him dad. He's really cool. He just told me that he had a brother who was a shrink, who got really close to a patient. The patient then killed himself, and so the shrink, Matt's brother did too, he was that upset. That's when Matt started to work with kids like us, to try to understand. I think his brother was fucked up and impulsively I told him, regretting it later from the look he gave me. But you can tell Matt is like that too. The day staff leaves at nine usually, but Matt will often stay till eleven or even later. On a good night, when no one is in restraint, he will stay until we are all asleep. Sometimes that will take until three in the morning.

MATT, DAD, MATT

He was the only staff member that had shown me his
own scars. We would compare each other's. His were
always bigger, no matter how many times I looked.

One was across his wrist. A failed attempted suicide he
had done when my age. He explained that cutting
across didn't work. You had to cut down along the
veins to succeed. The nurses would often tell him off
for this and he would answer with, "my kids know all
this already. It's not new to them." His other scars were
up and down his arms and legs. "I was a hooker," he
used to say knowing he would get confused looks.
What he meant was he used to work in the forest,
mauling wood, cutting down trees, and driving the
trucks with wood.

Often the tree trunks were hooked on to cables and
loaded. That job was called hooking. If the hook or
cable were to snap and break, down came the trunks.
The result is his scars. I think it was his wrist scar that
made him one of us. All the patients accepted him, but
not the other staff.

December 2000
I am in the class room now. We are watching a black
and white movie about Pearl Harbour. It's so boring; it's
like being back at school. A tec called Simon is taking
it. He was in some war. He is really cool though. He
almost got fired last week for giving Kaela and me
some sweets. The staff are so strict here, it's not like
we were going to give him head in exchange. I'd only
do that if he got us out of here. I hate it here. The glass
is bullet proof, the furniture, except the chairs, are
bolted down to the floor and they won't even let us
have pencils sometimes in case we stab each other. I
am still in scrubs. And still have to have a 24 hour even
though I've been here for ages.

A thirteen year old guy called Max got discharged
yesterday. He snorted all his meds that he had been

saving for ages, and they called code grey on him. All the Tec's came running with their rubber gloves, and the bed and put him in the time out room. Then they rolled him into an ambulance and took him to the hospital. A few hours later the Tec's took all his clothes and put them in a box. They said he was being transferred because he had done this too often. He was put in a maximum in his home city. The cleaners were called in to clean the restraint bed. Here the patients call it speedy. I hate it. It's cold and looks like the type hospitals use, except this one has the straps to hold you down.

The Professionals: I saw the psychiatrist there for ten minutes a week. If I didn't smile in our sessions I would get put on more medication. If I sighed my meds were doubled to twice the dose. The less I smiled the more I got. The more I got the less I smiled. I saw my therapist for one half hour a week. She dictated to me what I should say to my mother on the phone. She exaggerated what I told her about my parents. She misunderstood what I said in group therapy. I called her the rapist, because she raped me of what I talked about. She twisted and turned it until it was in her mumbled non-truthful words. I told her of a dream I had had of my mother trying to kill me. She told me it was a repressed memory that had once been real, than rang my mother to accuse her.

December 2000.
Ray got into another restraint today. He was in his usual time out room peering out of the window on the door, when all of a sudden, we saw him smear blood on it. I had never seen him do that before, but Kaela say's he does it a lot. No one including the staff knows how he does it. He has nothing on him. Brad says he bites into his wrists and just rips out his flesh. They called code red on him. Big Jared was on duty, and they got speedy in there. Ray was screaming for hours, and we were all laughing because he screamed really high pitched. The shots aren't as affective with Rob because his bodies used to them. The nurses say he

has been in places like this most of his life, and again wouldn't tell us his disorder.

When the nurses came out of the room, they were covered in blood, and dark red thick blobs. They left the room door half open. Ray was on the bed strapped down really tight. Then Debbie came out with two needles. I have never seen someone need two before. He has been in this room since I arrived. Come to think of it I have never actually seen the whole of Ray.

December 2000.
Ashley left today thank God! Ally tried to thump me last night, but I got to her first. We got into a big fight; luckily they didn't call code red. I don't know why, maybe because it was late. Matt was on duty, working late as usual, and carried me into the time out room. I was surprised he could carry me, especially as I was trying to bite him and was kicking and screaming like mad. Susan took Ally, who was muttering away to herself and shaking her head, to another seclusion. Matt was laughing at me and acting as if I was harmless. He then dumped me in on the floor and said when I had calmed down I could get my pillow and mattress. I was screaming and pacing the room, as he stood calmly by the door. He asked me why I was so pissed off and I told him about Ally. He asked me why I hadn't told him before and I said that she would have hurt me even more, he agreed.

Then he calmly told me that she was very disturbed for her age and she had a personality disorder. He said that she acts differently than other patients and that she will have it for the rest of her life. I was furious that she was a worse case than me and I started screaming loudly. The nurse came in and pulled him out. When they came back they said that they would restrain me if I didn't calm down. Matt then said he would deal with me. The angrier I got the more calm he acted. I move threateningly toward him and he sat down. I was shocked. I asked him what in the hell he was doing, he said he didn't want me to feel intimidated by him

50

standing up. That's when I started laughing. I mean he looked ridiculous. The nurse came in and gave me some pills to help me sleep. After a few minutes I got my pillow and tried to get some sleep. I was really upset but Matt sat beside me and held my hand. He told me his life story. I told him it was boring. He said he was trying to bore me to sleep.

Today when I woke up at lunchtime, Matt wasn't here. They said he had broken a staff-patient boundary and would not be working for a while. Usually staff cannot touch patients unless they have to, like in a restraint. There are exceptions though. Like when some one is very upset but not violent. Then a staff member can give them a hug, as long as it's in front of other people and the same sex. They say Matt might not come back just because he held my hand and it was in a closed room. I hate this place. Maybe I should hang myself when I get shoe privileges. That's when I am allowed to wear shoes, and the laces.

December 2000
Ally has been put back into the social ward, full time now. I don't see her unless their unit comes through ours to use the gym. She smiles at me and acts as if nothing happens. I just yell at her, and then she rolls up into a ball and cries like a baby.

I am finally out of the screamer and am back again with Kaela and a new girl called Lisa, from North West Academy, the school I was going to go to. Matt is back. He said he just needed to talk to some group of doctors and that was it. I think he was lying a bit so I didn't feel bad. I beat him six times at palace our favourite card game; then again he sometimes lets me win.

December 2000
Kaela and I have started mixing with a guy called Farley. He got sent here from juvenile hall. They didn't have space for him. He was sent there initially for stealing cars and dealing crack.

He is here for observation, to see if he has a mental disorder. The staff says he will be here for a few weeks. They are lying. I was sent here for observation for my voices, violence and hallucinations. I was meant to be here for a week before being sent to a maximum security school for nut jobs. I have been here months. He is huge; muscle wise. I have realised if I don't want to have guys constantly trying to rape me, I have to hang out with a certain group. Weirdly though this group contains some of the scariest cases.

In this group there is a guy called Brad. He has almost white hair that he used to die, so he has dark roots. He is really skinny because he thinks the staff are trying to poison him. He refuses to eat almost anything. He claimed in the last nut house he was in they tube fed him. He seemed really normal at first. Then one morning he put all his shit on his head. He had smeared it all over his face too. He was yelling in some language that no-one understood. The nurses said he thought it would stop people reading his mind. Kaela would tease him by going up to the screamers window and yell in that she could hear his thoughts. Every time she did it he would keep putting more shit on his head. He's now been transferred to adult psychiatric.

Then there is Kevin who is 15 and doesn't say much. He thinks there are know bones in his wrists, ankles and neck. None of us can figure out what disorder he has. He is funny and cool, but flips out if anyone touches him.

Then there is Davie, who is about 17 and is really cute. He thinks he is possessed. He has a very violent side to him that I have not seen but have heard about. He doesn't have emotions like normal people do. It is like he doesn't feel them. His foster parents are trying to get him taken out of this place. He is always twitchy with nerves, as he's never been put in a place like this before. He is usually put in jail but he is here for court reasons. I think it's a bit like observation. Also there is Angie. No one talks to her. She is 15 and like Ray, has been locked up most of her life. She is extremely weird. She is always sweet and kind of shy. She has a baby called Lana. She has curly black hair and is a doll. I'm serious she believes that this fucking doll is real. She feeds her and everything. The staff would take the doll away, but then she threatens suicide and screams her head off. She always stares at me and smiles for ages. I yell at her to look somewhere else, it creeps me out so much. The sweet over friendly people in horror movies are always the ones you should look out for. My god she is so scary. She walks like a floating ghost and always has her head tilted to one side. She is actually very pretty but looks seven years younger than her actual age because she is so petit.

December 2000

Now that I'm hanging out with Farley, I don't need to worry as much about the really violent patients. He controls them better than desperate doc. Farley is the one who decides when there should be a riot, or if some one should try stealing the master keys, which always fails. He tries to take down a staff member every other day.

He is always aggressive and violent. It is his anger that makes him irresistible. If he had been sensitive and caring I wouldn't be interested. For no reason he will flip and grab someone by the neck, or hold something to their stomach. It's usually a shank he has made out of something. He is nice though. He is not like other guys in here who think girls should be treated like shit. When I am with him no one touches me. He taught me how to sharpen the end of a biro pen he stole from the head nurse. It's now like a sharp plastic knife. He told me I could do it with a toothbrush and a comb too. He told me that dental floss is the worst and it can be really strong. He got put in time out today because he was pulling down on the hinge that is between a door and the wall. He reached up and just bent it out of shape as if it was jelly. He also taught me how to make really hard balls by getting lots of toilette roll and wetting it. He then rolled them up in balls and let them dry out.

When they are dry they are really hard. He threw some at AJ and they left huge welts on his back. He also taught me that to flood a toilet I shouldn't just put huge amounts of paper into the bowl but should roll some up into a ball and put it just inside the hole that drains the bowl. It really works! I spoke to my mom today. I was so excited! I haven't spoken to her for ages, but Linda my therapist kept telling me what to say. She said if I say anything bad about this place, or spoke Swedish she would disconnect the call. She had it on speaker phone so she could here everything. She is such a bitch. I asked Farley to jump her. He didn't answer me; I think he's going to think about it.

December 2000
I cut myself today. I did it with a comb and I loved it. It is amazing what you learn in here. I can now do it with my teeth, nails, and soul of my roommate's trainer. I am still restricted to just socks. I even taught myself to cut myself in a restraint. You just rub your arm against the strap over and over until the skin peels off. Like when you get a sore from a shoe from it rubbing, except bigger.

I am back in scrubs after being in my normal clothes for a day. It didn't feel good. I'm used to these now. I even had to put up a fight to get my hair band back. They cut my nails so short they bled. My leg still hurts from boot camp. It is numb in large areas from it being so wet and cold. They are sending me to the hospital tomorrow to get an x-ray. I don't know how they will transfer me. Not on foot or they know I'll run.

The Regular Staff: Many of the staff there were only a few years older than me, and were unqualified. They thought that their job was cool and something that they could tell their friends about. There were a few who would take the job seriously though, and who genuinely enjoyed it. Some helped me, some did not. Some abused me, some did not. Some had a real understanding of the pain I was in where as other staff members didn't grasp the idea of who I was. They didn't and couldn't understand me. That made them scared. People I find are always afraid of what they don't understand. In a nut house this turns to hatred, and hatred turns to abuse. But you learn to accept this. It was the staff that really cared who made the difference. They made everything bearable.

December 2000
I spoke to my mom again. My therapist dictated what I should say to her. I want to go back to England really badly. I hate it here so much. I'm finally in the bedrooms again, with Kaela. I had been in the time out room for longer than usual. My voices have been getting worse now. They say I talk to them with out realising, and that I will sit for a while and just stare at a wall. They say it's called disassociating.

We are on unit shut down. We can't leave our rooms because there have been too many restraints. We have been on unit shut down for four days now. It's so boring. They have even taken our mattresses so we can't sleep during the day. Kaela is throwing up and Lisa is biting her arm.

The x-ray went o.k. They put me on speedy in the time out room and gave me two shots. Then they rolled me into a van. When we arrived they put me into a wheel chair and strapped my arms and ankles to it. I was feeling terrible though. As if I was drunk. Every thing was in slow motion. I must have looked like a mass murderer. I was drooling and moaning because of the meds. Two big men in scrubs and a female nurse escorted me. The patients and visitors of the medical hospital pretended not to look, but I thought they acted hysterical. The more I laughed the more they looked, the more I laughed. Mothers guided their children to the other side of the room and junkies waiting for their scripts cheered. They thought I was an important nut patient. I wasn't.

I then went into the machine. When I woke up I was back here. They said they didn't know what was wrong with my leg but were going to get a physiotherapist.

THE 24 HOURS

To be a 24 hour nurse was not popular. Their job was to sit, listen and stop us trying to hurt ourselves or others. I always had the same three. There was Kristy, who every one thought was too young and too pretty to be working with fucked up kids. She was sweet and quiet, but if you ever crossed her you would know how she got the job. For her size she was the strongest woman I had ever met and was one of the best restraint technicians on the unit.

There was Wayne, a guy in his early twenties, with the face of a sixteen year old, who had more kids than I could ever remember. He would never blink but seemed to constantly stare. This gave him a weird appearance to the point many parents thought he was a patient. He also had a non-impressive permanent hard on, which he would explain, whilst sighing, was a medical condition and that he was on medication for it. There was also Matt who most of us called dad. A round yet muscular guy in his late forties who went round saying he had 26 children: us. He was my favourite. He had an addiction to card games and would challenge anyone to beat him. He was the only one who actually listened to you. And it wasn't with impatient eyes that constantly looked at the clock. "When hearing a problem or concern, time stands still and your only concern is to not patronise, not embarrass and not ignore the patient," he would often say. I always answered with, "You're good psychiatrist material." he was the only one who could usually get me to calm down and the funny thing was he didn't do anything. No restraint, no meds, no shouting or warning…. Just listening…

December 2000
I am so bored. There is nothing to do but play cards
with Matt and a young guy called Wayne, who has a
permanent hard on. I hope that big Jared isn't coming
in tonight. He doesn't let us play cards. It's Christmas
soon. It's so depressing here. There is loads of snow
outside. It must be freezing. It is cold in here too
though. We are only allowed five very thin hospital
blankets but I have eight. If they catch me they will get
really pissed.

Ray's time out room is right next to ours. He keeps
banging a tune with his head and Kaela and I have to
guess what song it is. It's the last resort for not flipping
out. Farley's room is across the corridor from ours. He
keeps showing off all his tattoos. A.J is doing a
sculpture with the paper water cups. He will build
something then knock it down, and then do it over. He
has his tongue pierced and keeps trying to find
something to put in it to keep it from closing.
He finally discovered a part of a comb that he put in
there. He is constantly trying to pierce or fuck
something. Farley and he share a room and he is
always trying to give Farley head.

December 2000
It is Christmas day and every staff member has put
something on our paper tree, but it's fairly plain
anyway. Matt and Simon put presents under it and we
all got something. They bought them with their own
money. That was kind of cool. We got rubber balls and
electronic games. However the staff confiscated the
balls because Farley threw them at Jack and A.J.
Farley was the first to be in a restraint today. It took
seven Tec's to take him down. He was only in it for five
hours though. We all got to sleep in an hour today
though I didn't feel the difference. I'm really depressed
lately and so am sleepy a lot of the time. With the extra
hour we all got up at eight instead of seven a.m. and
we get to go to bed at eleven pm, instead of ten pm.
We are usually so tired; I doubt anyone will be able to
stay awake till then.

Jack was restrained at lunchtime. We had to sit through his wailing. I am still restricted from the cafeteria, as always, so a few others and I had to stay behind. Ray was allowed out as a special treat. He is getting better. He usually just spends the nights in seclusion now.

Jack is one of the one's who screams the most. He sounds as though he is being murdered. It is horrible. If he doesn't shut the fuck up soon, I will do it for him, I swear…

CHRISTMAS DAY

He lay there, as if dead. Eyes glassed over, hair wet with sweat, body lifeless and ridged. His mouth open, his head tilted to one side, held down by a red restraint strap and buckle. A white cloth spread out under his chin, to soak up the constant dribble that leaked from his tongue. His bare arms revealed blue veins from where the straps were cutting down his circulation. His body jerked every few minutes, as if trying to refuse the drugs that had been injected into him. A patch of light, which had escaped through the bars on the window, settled on his cheek. This was the only beam of sun in that dark room.

A mental health technician, Brent, sat on a plastic chair behind his head, and was mumbling some thing religious into Jack's ear. Brent was bent over him slightly, stroking his shoulders gently, and occasionally switching the stained cloth for a new one. Every so often he would shine a light into his pupils to see his response.

The mill area was silent. I sat at the thin, cheap fold out table with my sandwich. This was my Christmas dinner. Most of the patients on youth acute were in the hospital cafeteria enjoying a warm turkey. Not me. Not the few that sat around me. The "c" sections they called us. The suicide risks, the rapists, the severely mentally ill kids, and me, whoever I was. I seemed to be tattooed

58

with a new label every week. I glanced around the depressing room. My fellow peers eating their food with their hands. Scooping up their soggy coco pops with their fingers. Apparently a plastic spoon was out of the question. I let my eyes drift to the snow, I couldn't play in. Then over to the phone I couldn't use. I thought of the box of clothes I'd been sent, which now lay in some storage locker. Apparently my behaviour restricted me to hospital scrubs. "Great Christmas," I thought, sarcastically…."Just great…."

The Other Patients: Most patients in there had a mental disorder of some type. On the unit I was in the ages ranged from twelve to seventeen. There were a lot of bulimics and anorexics. There were a few alcoholics and almost every patient had a drug history. Most of the male and female patients were aggressive and violent. The males often showed this by physically hurting others where as the females would usually resort to self-harm. They would take out their frustration on themselves. One or two patients in my unit had auditory or visual hallucinations. The majority had tried suicide at least once in their life. Many had been sexually and physically abused. Some had carried this out on younger siblings or classmates. There were one or two who had more severe problems and were there for trying to kill their parents or other people, but they were less common.

I didn't remain in contact with any, as I didn't have time, when leaving, to get their addresses. It is something that I regret. I have heard rumours that three patients on my unit finally were released on their eighteenth birthday and all three succeeded in committing suicide. One girl, my home girl, went back to heroin and prostitution. A good friend, a male patient, is now still in a very secure unit in New York and will probably be there for a good couple of years. However his release is certain it will just take a while and he is in good caring hands. I miss all of them still and I often think of them. They might not have been normal but they were

59

there for me in their own ways when I needed them. They were my friends.

December 2000
I'm so pissed off!!! I got restrained again yesterday. I hate them so much. Some patients like them but I don't. They are so annoying, and you feel really groggy afterward. I am in the screamer now. The others are in the mill area watching three movies as a special privilege. Ray keeps appearing at the window and trying to make me smile by pulling faces. Kaela also appeared at the window with Farley but then big Jared shouted at them, and they left.

Matt would come in a few times to shine a torch in my eyes and check my pulse. Simon smuggled me two chocolates. He told me, "to not give in to the enemy," He is such a war freak. Last night everyone watched loads of movies, and we were all allowed one bagel each. I'm pissed off I missed that. I can't even remember when I got to watch a film. It's strange but when a movie is on it's the only time every one settles down.

I hate feeling like this. Tomorrow I'm going to try to kill myself, but I will probably not get my shoelaces for a while. I have only been able to wear socks for weeks because I cut myself with my trainer. I rubbed the sole against my arm and took off patches of skin. I think it is because of friction or something. You just rub and rub away and it comes off in small crumb like bits. It's amazing what you can learn in here. When I get home I'm going to try it with sand paper.

THAT TAINTED ROOM

It smells of madness, it screams of madness, it contains madness. It also creates it. Within it I have nothing to do but face myself. I despise its existence.

This room like a mirror reflects my portrait. I cannot choose what I want to see. I am forced to except the fact I need it. That it takes bullet-proof glass and bolts to keep me from the world and sedation to keep me from myself. To calm the silent ticking bombs inside me. It does the opposite. It speeds up the dials, it pulls at the trigger. If I explode I do it away from scared patients and visiting families. From anyone's knowledge but the staff and me.

These four walls echo a language that only we can understand, we who know its pain, we who have lived within its grasp. I now know the language fluently. I will not let it hold me. I will not give in to its tempting. That tainted room twists my mind. I realise I can't get out. It has me rotting and drugged. Crying and tearing. My nails are ripping at its walls that do not peel or crack. Throwing my body at the window in its door that refuses to break and let me out.

And after endless attempts to release my anger, and when the drugs take effect, the only thing hurt in that room is me. My knuckles peeling, my wrists and fingers cracking, my sanity breaking. And yet still it contains me.

January 2001
Some patients had visitors today. Farley's mum came. His daughter came too. She's called Angel and is so cute. She had his dark hair that was really long, and she wore a little leather jacket. Her arms were covered in fake tattoos. She was going round saying, "what's up?" to every one. I think that's all she could say. She kept showing off some Disney character she had on her t-shirt. Farley was surprisingly gentle with her, and she got really upset when she had to go. He must have had her really young. She is two years old and Farley's parents have been helping him look after her. Angel's mother is apparently twenty years old and is in jail. Farley's parents talk to her in another language and she calls Farley pappi.

Ray's family came. He hadn't seen them for months. It was his mom, and two sisters. The third sister didn't come because of what he did to her. It's no wonder he is so feminine, being around women all his life. When we are bored he will tuck his dick between his legs and paint his nails with the board marker. He will then go up to big Jared and yell, "Who's your bitch?!" Then, Big Jared replies by yelling, "SECLUSION NOW!"

His mom was yelling at him. Saying things like he was a little sex pervert, that his sister was in the protection system and that he would go to hell. She then broke down and was asking God why she spawned such a wicked son. I was laughing. It was all her fault. She used to beat him, and make him take baths in really hot water when he was little. Apparently she was trying to cleanse him. She is such a religious freak. So he sat with me the whole afternoon. He thinks about sex 24 hours of the day and has molested kids but he is sweet. Like the fucked up little brother I never had. The difference with Ray is he doesn't know it is wrong, so you can't blame him. He wasn't like the other sick guys. He hardly ever knows where he was let alone what he had done. He looks kind of funny too. He sucks his thumb all day long, so his two upper front teeth stick out. He also has an annoying freckle just below his right eye.

Jack's mom came. He was so nervous that Debbie, the nurse in charge, wrapped him up in a blanket and hugged him. That was a rare sight, though I don't know why. Most of us need hugs to calm us down, not meds though we would never admit it and never get them. Jessica got to go out with her parents and a 24-hour. Angie, A.J, Kaela, Cameron and some others including me didn't ever get visitors. We each had our reasons, and we didn't like to discuss them.

January 2001
I'm really pissed off. I was in the gym room doing the boring exercises for my bad leg with slime ball Tad. Usually he goes on about how youths in nuthouses

deserve to be there but today he was being overly nice. I told him I was sick of him fucking feeling me because I felt disgusting. All the staff here wear these alarm buttons round their necks and I pressed his.

The nurses and Tec's came running. Before I could say anything they grabbed me and took me to seclusion. I am so fucking angry. I've cut my self really bad but I don't remember when, or how. Tad was told never to come back; in case I hurt him. It's a fucking joke. I tried to talk to the staff here but they won't listen. At least he is fired. Someone is coming to ask me about it, I might have to fill in a form.

THE PHYSIOTHERAPIST

He put one hand inside my pants. His skin dry and sharp against my soft hospital scrubs. He didn't play though. His eyes locked onto mine. He started rubbing hard, round and round. I lay limp and ridged, like dead. I heard his breathing increase to a raspy grunting. It was thick with mucus, hot and heavy. His free hand clamped down over my mouth. I wondered how I must have looked to him then. I wondered whether I would get a bruise in the hollow of my cheek and across the bone, where his thumb dug in. My mind was blank.

I could feel my eyes swelling with angry tears. His face so close to mine. His sharp frame became blurred. I frantically blinked. I was trying to focus, squinting to see him. I wanted to scream. I wanted to run. Hide under a blanket in the warmth of someone's arms. I didn't. I let him do it. He carried on. Faster, harder, his fingers were cutting my skin. A fierce nail was getting caught. My cheeks burning, like sunburn from the tears. An eternity passed. I pressed the emergency button on the cord round his neck.

Then there was shouting. Staff came running. His eyes bulging in hatred and still I lay there. While frozen in time. It felt good. To see a man once so powerful, shake like a rabbit. He was a terrified animal. A stain

63

forming on his wall mart pants. His cum was spreading. His hand was covering it.

January 2001.
I have just fucked Farley. He managed to get past the security mirrors and across the corridor without getting caught. He fucked Kaela first which was strange, I thought she was les. The Tec's came in soon after and we all had our privileges taken away. They didn't know too much though. The staff had come to the conclusion to the fact that he had not had the time to do anything else. They are so dumb. I took a shower with a 24-hour in the room. They are watching me more closely now. I scrubbed my body so hard that I have freckly bruises all over. I feel dirty.

My voices are back and are really bad. I had gone about three days with out them. The hallucinations are back again too. I have been disassociating again without noticing. The staff put ice-cubes in my hands when I do it. They say it helps me to come back, from that place I go. It kind of shocks me back into reality. It is better than being injected. I wish I could remember. It must be better than here.

FARLEY

He was bigger than I thought. My back turned to him. My knuckles dug into the wall. His hipbones were knocking. Every muscle in his face clenched. All I could think about was why I had to have sloppy seconds. He pushed further, before he settled into a rhythm. I could feel a stabbing pain just below my belly button. I thought the skin there would burst. I felt as though I was giving birth to some alien creature who refused, and kept clawing its way back in.

I could see his reflection in the mirror. It was evil and nasty. Grunting and gasping for air. His eyes were clamped shut, as if desperately shutting out his own image. One hand, permanently glued to my right hip. The other one was over my own left hand. He was

64

crushing my bones further into the wall. I felt the skin on my knuckles break and burn.

I saw him cum. Every muscle in his olive face was hard and tight. He looked ugly and desperate. Like a withering flower. The glued hand started thumping my lower back. Just above the crack in my bum. He withdrew and collapsed to the floor. His chest was heaving. His hair was sticky with sweat. I glanced at the wall. Red smudges of blood. They were watery and fake. I felt the muscles squeeze his cum out of me. It dribbled and ran down my leg like period blood.

The neon bathroom light flickered. There was an impatient knock at the door. He pulled up his pants, and then knelt on his knees. Then a burst as they rushed in. Arms behind his back they led him away. I smiled and so did he.

January 2001
I'm on level 'C' again. It's the lowest of the low. No privileges, no sharps, no nothing. There were two 24-hours with me all the time. I have been in too many restraints and have cut up my arms and legs so badly that they have put me in the time out room permanently. I hope I won't be here for months. Ray is finally in the bedrooms now. His roommate's are planning on raping him tonight. Well that's the word around here. Farley says he won't watch Ray's back, "you rape, you get raped," he always says.

Ray was in here for ages before they let him out. I'll go crazy, well crazier if they do that to me. I don't like the walls in here. They make me dizzy. They are a horrid, sickly hospital green. They are so plain, and yet you can see your past and future in them in quick flashes that come and go.

Chris the drug therapist keeps telling me that I am an alcoholic, just because I fucked guys for drink. I think that I drank because I was down or in a binge, but not because I was addicted. Not that anyone listens to my opinion or anything.

My head hurts today. A.J. and I tried to get behind the nursing station to get something, anything, and big Jared came and slammed our heads down on the counter. I swear he can't do that. We complained and then he came and had a word with us and said we shouldn't waste the nurse's time with fake complaints. Every one knows big Jared does stuff that he is not supposed to. And he only does it to the severe cases. The ones he knows he can get away with. He once restrained me for holding a crayon the wrong way. He once restrained Cameron because when he needed a piss sample, Cameron said he just couldn't go. Any excuse is good enough for big Jared to take advantage of his position.

February 2001
Desperate doc is such a dick. My 24-hours need to be in the room with me but not to actually stare at me when I shower. He has labelled me, obsessive compulsive disorder, addict, and possible split personality. I think he is nuts. I can't possibly have all those at the same time. The words fucked up I understand but not the others. He won't even explain to me what they mean. He is such a cunt, I hate him.

I only see him for about five minutes every other week and he says that he records the sessions so that the patients can't accuse him of anything. I think that that's total bullshit, and that he says it to scare us. He is evil. He never listens and is really patronising. If you ask him why he works with fucked up kids, he will say, "the money, there's know point lying." what he means is from this job he gets a lousy pay check, but some private patients parents, will pay him a fortune to personally collect there kids to bring them here and to see them every day. He doesn't give a fuck about anyone of us.

He knew about the physiotherapist, and about big Jared, and he doesn't do anything. I am never going to trust a psychiatrist again. They all want your money, or to fuck you or to hurt you. To watch you squirm under their power. If you say anything aggressive to him, or complain he will just put you on more meds. If I ever saw him on the outside I might well consider killing him. I know I'm not the first to think this and I know I won't be the last

MOVIES

On Saturdays we got to watch a movie in the mill area. This was a rare treat that I rarely got to join in on. Those in the time out room didn't get privileges. But if you sat by the door you could just make out the words they were saying. When they put you in the time out room, usually you'd be out in four days. By then you'd be "Rested." I always used to scream, "I'm going on a holiday see you in a week," when they put me in there, which was a lot.

The movies they showed made me wonder just how fucked up the staff were. We'd see films like, 'One Flew over the Cuckoo's Nest', and 'Girl Interrupted'. They only put everyone in a bad mood, and gave others ideas, strange. They wouldn't show 'Trainspotting' or 'Requiem for a Dream' in a rehab, or would they?

February 2001
My mom's coming in a week! Jessica hung herself a few nights ago with the laces of her shoes in the shower. I'm so angry. She stole my idea! Kaela and I found her. They called code grey. They cleaned all her stuff out. It was weird though, our day didn't stop. The nurse's said change is bad and that not going on with our routine would ruin everything. We did have a group on it though. That was really sick. Farley and Kevin were joking about it, like it was funny. I didn't say anything. Not a lot of girls did.

The site wasn't like you would think it would be. Her face wasn't in a twisted position, she didn't smell. She didn't look like you are supposed to when you're dead. Kaela had shoved my hand on her cheek. It didn't feel dead. Then again I don't know what it is supposed to feel like. It freaked me out. Ray said that when some people die, their extremities go blue.

It wasn't until later that a nurse told us she wasn't dead when we found her but more passed out. I think she died later in the hospital. It's a shame; I was so excited at the thought that I had touched a dead person. I knew she looked too well. Every night since then I have had nightmares of me touching her face and then she would suddenly open her eyes. They are horrifying. I'm trying to block it all out, so I can deal with it another time. That's what I always do when I don't want to remember. Matt says that's part of my problem.

The thing I've noticed most about the kids in here is that they don't react like they are supposed to. I didn't realise till my shrink told me that I should have flipped out when we found her. He said normal kids don't laugh. They cry. It's true. No one I know on the outside would have acted like we did. They would have needed therapy for years. To us it was nothing. Tomorrow it will be old news. Does the fact that death does not scare me make me fucked up?

Farley got really mad today. I think it was because of Jessica, but he wouldn't admit it. The weird thing was although some of us were sad, most of us were jealous. Jessica had succeeded in something that the majority of us had tried and failed, or did not have the balls to do. We were put in the gym while the Tec's tried to take him down.

They are thinking of giving me liquid meds in case I cheek them. The nurses say that when things like this happen, it gives patients ideas. The head nurse told me that although most patients go on about suicide it very rarely happens on the ward. If it happens it is usually a couple of months after they go home. If I wanted to die, I wouldn't do it in a nuthouse where they have a hospital next door, to pump it out of you. Or those horrid shots they give you that force you to puke it all up, and that create a stinging deep down in your Stomach. The voices are back. I wish they would go away.

THE MUSIC MAN

Twice a week we woke to his playing. He would sit at the nursing station, lean back in his chair, face the long corridor where our rooms were and play his guitar. He would lift his right leg slightly to get a better grip. Some times we would hear his identification badge that hung on a cord round his neck, clank against the wood if he leaned over.

He came to work early. Long before the day staff would arrive. When they did he had to stop playing. They were not fond of his music. If I was up early or couldn't sleep I would look out of my bedroom window into the parking lot. Then I would see his old car drive up. It was always dirty and loud. The sun would never be up but it was still light enough to see outlines. He would take out the case from the boot, and every time it looked like a body in a duffle bag. I would always scare the new patients by telling them that that was what happened if you pissed him off.

The night times were the worst. After several restraints and kids screaming or crying, it was calming to wake up to his playing. Every thing was quiet then. Even the loud patients who were sad shut up just for half an hour to listen. We would lie awake in our cold beds and pray that the day staff would crash on the way to work, so we could have a few more minutes. Just a little while longer before the reality of where we were would come flooding back.

We called him the music man. I never actually knew his real name. Most patients didn't. It would have been so disappointing if we realised his name was Fred. We didn't want to know that he was human, or that he perhaps lived an ordinary life. We wanted him to always be the mysterious music man we thought of him as, and wanted him to be. He new simple cords and always used the same ones. Occasionally he would use the nursing desktop counter as a drum.... but never loudly.... His playing was always soft, quiet, and gentle. Often he would also sing. His songs were sad and low. He sung about love, he sung about his losses and he sung about his life. He sung about us too. About our fear and our hate, our emotions and our problems. He took all our horrid pain that was kept secret within the surrounding hospital walls, all our endless disgusting agony and turned it into something beautiful with the flick of a thumb.

February 2001

Oh! My God, my mom is here! This is so cool. Right now she is in with my shrink, who all of a sudden seems charming. I am sitting in Chris's room and I don't even have a nurse with me. I am on 15 minute checks, but the fact that I don't have some one staring at me all the time is so cool. I can't remember the last time when I was on my own. Never, since I came in here.

She looked really scared when she saw me. When I left home I had really long hair. Then at boot camp they shaved it off. I knew she was coming this morning, just not what time. I was so nervous I was sick all along the corridor. It was really cool to see her. She had got me coke and a pizza. I ate it so fast. Anything hot, alone was great. But my stomach wasn't used to it or so much that I threw it up hours later, and got diarrhoea from the caffeine in the coke.

We get fed here small amounts. Not to the point that they starve us but to the point that everyone who first arrived needed at least two weeks, to get used to the amounts. They are inconsistent. One day you would get massive meals that you are forced to finish. The next day you are given, bread, fruit and salad. I'm only allowed sandwiches and cereal. I am restricted to finger foods. I can't even use a plastic spoon in case I hurt someone with it.

There was a restraint in progress when my mom came back to Chris's room. Wayne ran in to the room to explain every thing was o.k. It was Farley. He later said he was trying to prove to my mom that these things happened. She looked very worried. We couldn't see it but could hear it just outside the door to the room.

February 2001
I think my dad is going to try and get me out of here. My mum said she would try. At first they wouldn't even let her come see me. She left a few days ago. She said it would probably take three to four weeks. I can't wait. A.J said he is going into a private clinic in a month, and Farley is going to adult psychiatric in Queens, New York in 28 days, as he will soon be turning eighteen. I guess he doesn't need to go to jail after all. I feel sad that I am going to have to say goodbye to home girl Kaela. She will most likely go back to the nut school or her stepmother's place in Chicago. Her stepmother is a dancer and is dating a guy half her age.

My mum said I'm either going to go to The Priory in Roehampton or The Cromwell Hospital in London. I thought it sounded strange that I wasn't going to be put in a nut house. That's where I belong, isn't it? Then again it might be a locked ward.

Departure: On leaving the nut house, I felt sad. I had found my home, my place in the world. This is who I am; this is where I belong, and where I should stay. I am one of these nuts. I am not normal. It is here where I fit in. I didn't want to be thrown out to that world that would judge me. Where everyone covers up their scars and paints a smile on their faces. I did not know how to live there, nor do I now. I am not ready, I never will. It was safe in the hospital. It was safer than the world outside. In here I worried about suicide. I can handle

71

that. But to worry about bills and buying food, I cannot. I felt helpless. I didn't feel safe. I didn't want to leave. Once you have tasted hell you can't let go.

HELL EXISTS

It wasn't fun in there. There were the times when some one managed to kill themselves, or when we had to fall asleep to the wailing of some one in a restraint. Most nights you would have to fall asleep to crying and screaming, night times were the worst. That's when the occasional riot would start, and unit shut down would begin. Or when you woke to some one either trying to get into your bed and into your pants or trying to hurt you because they thought you were a government agent plotting against them..... Like when a staff member hurt a patient and got away with it, or having inspections by the medical board asking you questions and knowing that if you told them something the staff would find out.

Most patients got out before they turned eighteen. A lot were passed on to mental wards in their hometowns. Some went to boot camp, others to Adult Psychiatric. Some were on the Acute Unit for weeks others for years. And although I hated it there it was scary to leave. In the world outside people didn't understand what it is like to want to die or you just flip out for a while. In a place where perfect is desired the weird and mad are condemned. Normal, happy people don't understand what its like to want to cut into your flesh, or to hear voices all day. I now understand why the few patients, who did kill themselves, did it when they had left. When they realised they could not live or ever be part of this world.

February 2001
Well I'm finally out. I am sitting in a hotel in Seattle. My dad is in a room next door. I'm so paranoid. I made him take everything sharp in the room, and even a lamp and also a hair dryer. What am I going to do with that? Blow my hair to death. Oh right, water, electricity. I

think it is because I have been in such a safe environment and now it's too much to suddenly be thrown in at the deep end in a place that is full of objects that I can hurt myself on.

NIBH has given me meds until I get to the new place. I laid them all out on the bed crushed them and snorted them; otherwise I won't be able to sleep. Whenever I do this I keep thinking that spiders are on me. They should kick in soon. If I don't take them I will keep having images of Jessica or my voices will get louder. I can't handle that tonight.

I have a king size bed, but I am going to sleep on the floor. I'm not used to sleeping without the familiar plastic sheets. I have a TV with 105 channels but I'm not going to watch it. I feel strange and unhappy. I wish somebody would open my door with a flash light and whisper checks. I want Big Josh to yell lights out, and hear Rob knocking on the wall. I don't hear any screaming. It's too quiet. It doesn't feel right.

I miss all my nutty friends at the hospital. I couldn't wait to leave, but it's scary in the real world. Here I have to hide my scars and if I flip out at my voices, like in the hotel lobby, I have to pretend I saw a mouse. I searched for people like me, but found only smiling tourists and businessmen. I feel out of place.

There were no secret smiles of understanding, no distant eyes that saw what I saw, no twitching youth who new where I had been. I want to crawl back into my world of blackness, my hospital; where I am understood. There was nothing; just me, a smudge in a picture perfect world.

My View on the Place: I do not know to this day if I should have been in a mental hospital. Some say I should have, others disagree. Now that I know I am a borderline I don't feel it was necessary. Then again who knows how far I would go to hurt someone. If I had been a danger to others or even myself, then yes. But at that time in my life I don't think I was. I feel that for a lot of people they can provide a healthy and safe place where their needs can be met. In any hospital I now have learnt that there is only so much that the staff can do. The rest is up to the patient. If someone does not want to get better then they won't. I believe if I need a hospital like this in the future then it would be good for me. As long as the staff know how to deal with patients like me then it is good. If it is safe and run properly then it can help someone like me greatly. The hospital I went to has supposedly been shut down now due to neglect and abuse. However there are several safe and secure units out there that do not act like many of these hospitals that you hear about. I feel there is a lot of negative thoughts and rumours surrounding them, but this is usually from people that have never had first had experience with them.

How It Affected Me: I did connect with many patients in there. I think now that this was because of the fact that it had been the first time in my life that I had been with other teenagers who had similar difficulties to me. I could relate to every single patient in some way or another. At that particular point in my life I didn't know or understand my disorder. It was because of this that I just presumed that I was crazy, so obviously deep down thought I needed to be there. Even though when I was there I hated most of it, I still sometimes miss it. I have an occasional nightmare about abuse or the feeling of being locked up. But at the end of the day I have to think of it as a positive experience that taught me a lot of lessons about other people as well as myself. And although I would never wish a friend or family member to have to experience what I did, if I needed it in the future I would go. Maybe kicking and screaming all the way. But I would go. I have accepted that because of who I am, there might come a time again where a mental hospital is the only thing that will keep me alive.

CAN YOU SEE?

Can you feel my pain?
Can you see my scars?
My body's down on earth,
My minds among the stars.

CRAZY BOY RAY

Sitting in his locked room,
Where he has been for a while,
Blood smeared on the window,
Tears in his sorrow filled eyes.
Starring out smiling,
Trying to understand,
Why he is so disturbed,
From young girls he is band.
He taps the glass for attention,
To anyone who passes by,
Spending most nights banging his head,
In the day all he does is cry.
Once he was innocent,
But his upbringing made him bad,
Now he sits in that locked room,
Knowing he is mad.
He does not know his identity,
Sexual fantasies play in his mind,
And you can't help but like him,
Though he was a child rapping a child.

DEATH WISH.

They roll you in with flashing lights,
The nurses prick you without care,
Only on TV have you seen this sight,
Other patients turn to stare,
Shouting, panic then it starts,
Junior doctors with sweaty palms,
Bleeping machines monitor your heart,
Holding stomachs, there first self-harm,
Heavy padding on your fragile wrists,

For years so lonely now the final end,
But a dance with death it has a twist,
Calls to family, calls to friends,
Stitches urging your skin to heal,
Ward doctors smiling to reassure,
This isn't happening, it isn't real,
Do they not realize there is no cure?
Angry frowns, your wasting their time,
The rubber snaps, the gloves come off,
Machine is silent, just a flat line,
Some are silent, others scoff,
Professionals analyse, young nurses sob,
They should be happy with your wish,
Doctors swear, "Fuck these nut jobs,"
Now your dead are you missed?
Family are shocked and sad,
You realise now that you're gone,
Friends that said your mind was bad,
They were right and you were wrong.

SOME ONE!

Some one hear me before it is too late!
I'm trapped in my emotions,
And I'm trying to escape,
Someone help me!
My body I have to sacrifice,
But to feel alive,
I have to pay the price,
Someone save me!
I'm standing by the ledge,
Will anyone reach me?
Or will I step over the edge,
Someone stop me!
For I am not in control,
Maybe this is the answer,
Will death make me whole?

DISSASOCIATING

I don't know what I've done,
I don't know what I've seen,

I don't know what I've said,
I don't know where I've been.
I'm sitting on the floor,
How long has it been this time?
I'm feeling dazed and confused,
Am I loosing my mind?
The last thing I remember,
The time was about 2:00,
I'm covered in someone's blood,
Has an hour passed, or a few?
This blood must be mine,
But my cuts and wounds are dry.
I've probably been here for ages,
I don't even know why!
I don't know what I've done,
I don't know what I've seen,
I don't know what I've said,
I don't know where I've been.

WINGS

I wish I could grow wings,
Then I would fly,
Out of my cage and start a new life.
Our hell has no name,
Our hell has no face,
With affection I leave my self sliced.
This dark hole is cruel,
A place just for rules,
And forever we will serve our sentence,
Our fear is too great,
We don't cry but we scream,
And all that we own is resentment.
They have tools of punishment,
The shots and the straps,
And none is favoured the most,
Used for their protection,
They erase our recollection,
Our memories haunting like ghosts.
I wish I could grow wings,
Then I would fly,
Into the world I once tasted.

But if granted the chance,
With my demons I'd dance,
For my mind is already wasted.

PSYCH WARD RESTRAINT.

Here I lie dying,
Here I lie crying,
Lying here I try to pretend,
I scream,
I shout,
Yet I still have no doubt,
That like this my short life will end.
Here I lie bleeding,
Here I lie needing,
Hoping that some one will save me,
In this life,
In this state,
If I'm fucked up I debate,
The answer I come to is maybe.
Here I lie twitching,
Here I lie itching,
I've been lying here for so long,
I can see,
I can hear,
But still I'm in fear,
Why was my mind born so wrong?

CHAPTER THREE

London-1 Hospital.

March-April
17 years old

Arrival: When I arrived I was shocked. I sat with my bag on a posh looking chair while waiting to see the nurse. My mother was with me and was scanning a leaflet she had picked up down stairs at the front desk. A man with a ponytail introduced himself and showed me to my room. He was not wearing gloves. No bruises to show he had recently restrained someone. He was actually smiling. He didn't grab my arm to keep me from running. I didn't feel the need to. I wasn't that scared.

First Impression: There were no restraints! There were no time out rooms (that I saw.) it looked more like a hotel than a hospital. I had my own room and a bed that went up/down, forward/backward at the push of a button….And a TV…sky TV! I had my own bathroom. I am still not sure that this is an actual hospital.

I get to see my mum often in here. She only lives around the corner so she can come whenever she wants to during visiting hours. I did yoga today. I have never done it before but it was quite relaxing. The only bad thing about it was that it was really early in the morning and because I am on heavy sleeping drugs I am groggy until midday. I saw my sister a few days ago. It was so weird as I hadn't seen her for so long. She just ran up and hugged me and was so happy to see me. I got a bit bored though. All she did was talk about the boys in her life and her school. It was nice to hear about her life but she went on talking for about an hour. I got angry when she left. All she could think about was herself and not me. I am stuck in a hospital. I don't have the freedom that she has. Why does she have to tease me about her life outside these walls?

I don't want to hear about her perfect life. She was complaining about how hard her life was. There was a boy who she liked but who didn't seem to like her in return. I mean come on! That's hardly something to worry about. I wondered how she would like to be in my shoes for a while. Screaming voices in her ear and not being able to resist the razor and worrying that a patient might rape you when sleeping. It pisses me off that her biggest daily problems are her spots or shaving her legs. She doesn't seem to even begin to comprehend how hard my life is.

I'm debating suicide while she is debating what outfit to wear to a party. The worst thing is that she seems so much happier now that I am not at home. Since I went into hospital she gets all the attention at home. She really does seem more comfortable now that I am not around.

The Professionals: I saw my psychiatrist for the first time ten minutes after I had arrived. I then saw him almost everyday after that. He even saw me on bank holidays. I don't think I had a set time span with him. If I didn't have anything to talk about he would only stay five minutes, but when I had a lot to talk about he would stay much longer. He was the first psychiatrist that I actually started trusting. He was the only one who seemed to know me, the real me, my disorder that is. It took me a long time to realise that he had been right all along. I spent the future years trying to diagnose myself. I wanted to know who I was and why. He had the answer the whole time and I could have known too, if I had just asked. My therapist was a different story. I didn't really dislike her in anyway but at the same time there was nothing about her that I liked either. She would listen to me but wouldn't connect with much I said. Most sessions I had with her she used to sleep. She napped and I talked, until one of the nurses would come in to check up on me and she would wake.

BEING BORDERLINE

To be a Borderline is like having your period every day of the year. For me it is like having hundreds of different moods in just an hour alone. It is hell.

One minute I hate some one, the next minute I don't. Then I hate myself for thinking that I hate them. Then I hate them for making me feel this way. Then I hate myself for hating them for making me feel I hate them when I don't....and that is what it is like constantly, or at least at the bad times. When I am a bit more normal, I will obsess on why I am not thinking like that, until I have myself so worked up that I do start to feel like that, and then I will get angry that I started myself on this subject when I hadn't thought about it for so long.

Then I will obsess on why I haven't thought about it for so long, and so on it goes in a circle over and over until I collapse. Then while lying in a heap on the floor I think of why I do this all the time. It never stops unless I am doing well. In other words, unless I am stable and getting better.

At other times I will decide I need to get laid. I will go out and find a guy who likes to talk trash to girls. I will let myself get verbally abused for a while and then leave him. Then I will wallow in self-pity as to why poor little me is always stuck with shitty men. Not even realising I went in search for one. If I am with a guy who is sweet, funny, sensitive and generally prince charming, I will drive them away. I will cut myself, scream at them do anything possible for them to leave me. I think they can't handle me; I am not worth them so it would be best for me not to be with them. When they are gone I want them back.

I am only like that at my worst times, unfortunately that is often. It has been happening for several years at the very least. On top of that there are the voices. Unlike anything anyone else can understand or experience. They scream at me, they order me, they congratulate

81

me. Sometimes they are nice and quiet, other times they are nasty and very loud. If I am listening to music I can't hear them. I guess they don't have super powers as they claim. I could kiss the man who created walkmans. It would be a man wouldn't it?

They are annoying I could be having a good conversation with a dear friend and then they would start. I will start twitching my head or roll my shoulder in agitation. That friend won't call me or see me again.

The hallucinations are the worst. I call them the white people. I don't know why. I have seen them since I was six. People, well mostly doctors find that hard to believe. That is probably because it doesn't say so in a book. They will only believe things studied and written down in some professional's bible.

When I was young they were imaginary friends, now that I am older they are part of a disorder. They have long disfigured faces, and jet black hair. Their eyes are completely black and they are dressed in hospital gowns. There can be groups of thirty of them and then there can just be one. They don't have a sex and their voices are all the same.

When I was little they used to play hide and seek with me in the woods. I must have been a freaky child. They used to play nice games. They don't play those anymore. They taunt and they rave at me. They want me to do things. They threaten and they cry and howl. They scream and yet know one seems to hear them but me.

When I was six they were ones who urged me to rip out my teeth. I did with a metal hair clip. After I had taken out two at the back, and played with the blood in the bathroom sink I got bored and went to bed.

On top of all this there is the binge eating, vomiting, cutting, violent sex, wanting to die, more issues on men, not having a clue of who I am, losing moments of time-like black outs without the alcohol, and still there is more... And then some one has the audacity to tell me I deserve to live. If you lived my life you would understand wanting to die. You would wish me luck and hand me a kitchen knife.

Of course this is only at the bad times. When things are going good, or as good as it gets everything gets cut in half. But I am still dealing with some of my problems even at the best of times.

Imagine going through all this all day, every day. Imagine having a session with me. I reckon anyone who can put up with me, or even keep up with me for just half an hour every so often really does deserve a medal. I really am challenging, demanding and exhausting. Not just to myself but to those around me. And I wouldn't have it any other way.

The Regular Staff: The nurses on my unit were all nice enough. They were good at listening. If I didn't have anything to talk about then they would ramble on for hours at a time about their life. It was a relief sometimes to hear their problems concerning work and boyfriends rather then drugs and suicide. They rambled and I listened or vice versa. It was good to talk to them as it stopped me thinking of myself the whole time.

My dad came today. I was so angry with him. I have let him come and see me for the first time in ages and what did he do? He was asking me when I should go back to school. He wanted to know when I would get better and if I think I can start next September at a new school. He said I had exams to take and that I should speed up my recovery. Speed up my recovery?! Does he think that I can just flick a switch in my mind and then, bingo, I'm normal? I hate him. I am trying so hard not to cut and then he does this. No one seems to understand. I secretly want to die. I am planning my suicide and all he can talk about is the embarrassment to the family if I don't finish my education. I started to scream at him. Not words or sentences. I just screamed. I yelled until my lungs were sore. My voice was strained afterwards. All my emotions and anger came out all at once and I thought if I had a knife in my hands I would have killed him.

It scared me. The fact that I am so upset, that I don't care about hurting someone that badly is shocking. But I don't. I have nothing to lose. I don't care about my life why should I care about anyone else. The nurse has just given me some pills, their usual cocktail of pills that numb. I don't have the energy to cut. I feel as though years of not sleeping has now caught up with me and smacked me in the head. My body feels limp. My hands feel heavy. I've got to stop writing.

The Mistress-Sophie

I don't have the time or energy to worry about divorce and separation. Go fuck your mistress and tell her that you have chosen her over us, I am sure she will be proud of you. Lie there at night and know that our mother is dying on the inside and crying on the outside. That she hates you and still loves you at the same time. Go and play perfect families with her children and her dogs and promise us that our lives won't change or be that different than before. Convince us that changing schools, house and friends isn't that bad while you let her move into our home.

Let our house become an empty shell. It is too big to not have children running round it. Far too large for a couple and three dogs. Let it slowly lose its charm and warmth. The only home we really loved and its great big gardens that filled my mother's days for years. Now that it is all dressed up in her awful choice of fabric's and furniture, we don't want to visit the place where we grew up and became the people we are today. Your friends who attend your parties sigh at the memory of that a family home it used to be and talk of what it once was with such fondness that they dare not tell you. The gardens, the animals and the great flower

84

arrangements are all gone. They're all gone because you couldn't let us have two homes. You could have bought many more and yet you wouldn't. You had to take our home and our life away. The one we had just settled into. Now it is empty and always cold. A big English house dolled up in foreign fabrics here and there scattered with no love or interest.

Don't tell us how it is still our home and that we are welcome. Our rooms are now guest bedrooms and filled with things we have not chosen or wanted. Don't tell us how you are sorry for the way things worked out. Don't tell us how you miss us on holidays; you are preoccupied with her children now. Don't try and be interested in our lives now that you have her, you never bothered before.

One of the worst days of my life was when I met her. You introduced us without warning and then proceeded to dance with her all night in front of me and my sister. I swore I wished you dead a thousand times all night long. No one we knew could quite believe you did that.

Don't sit with friends and talk about her as if you have been married to her for years. It makes me sick to see old family friends so excepting of the two of you. You leave my mother several times. You fuck her friend behind her back and then finally put her out of her misery and divorce her. You are incredibly tight with the money you give her, even though both you and your mistress are loaded, and yet then everyone takes your side. They still invite you to parties and not my mother. They attend your shoots and birthday celebrations while leaving my mother alone. Not only does it make me want to spit on their graves once they are dead but I feel sorry for their children for having parents with such low morals that they pick sides with the richer friend. The one they never liked before when he was still married to my mother. How they can live with themselves is beyond my understanding. How can they laugh and joke with a man who has put his family through hell? How can they not call on my mother or invite her to anything? Jesus how can they be so selfish and not understand why she hasn't gotten over the worst thing imaginable?

I still haven't received an apology from the woman who had to fuck my father while he was still married. This is the woman who couldn't wait until she was divorced. This is the woman who was the cause for my final breakdown and entrance into a treatment centre. She was the one who caused a family to break up all because she couldn't keep her knickers on and didn't have a heart.

She can not possibly know how much by how many people she is hated and despised because of what she did. Because of what you both did. She hasn't seen what you were like when we were growing up. You were the nasty man who just shouted at us all the time, the man who spanked me because I was cheeky. You were the man who put his job first.

No you deserve each other, although my father will probably cheat on you too. I don't believe you were the first woman he slept with while he was married to my mother. I believe he moved us from London to Gloucestershire so that during the week he could do what ever he wanted without his family knowing. Well, that's Swedish men for you, isn't it? They all seem to wife swap and fuck around with each other. On my father's side of the family divorce rate and cheating is high. I hope that you are proud of yourself for making a ten year old cry herself to sleep knowing that her dad was with you and not her mother. Well done the pair of you! Great parenting skills!

My dad called today. He told me that my doctor had told him not to visit me. Dad sounded angry. He told me that no doctor should or could stop him seeing his own daughter. I laughed harder than I had in a long time. It was me that didn't want him seeing me again not my doctor. The fact that my doc doesn't fall for my dad's charm and manipulation skills pleases me even more. Usually everyone feels sorry for my dad. They think that he is such a good and caring father, who has always been there for me. Finally a doctor has realised he is full of shit. Caring and supportive is possibly the last thing that my father is. In my whole life he has been there for me for two things, discipline and money. He tries to control me. He can't and that makes him so angry. I don't care. Life is great without him. I can do what I want. I can be my own person. When my brother was my age he was living abroad. My dad was proud of this. I am still a baby in my dad's eyes. I cannot do anything that my brother did at my age, and it is down to the simple fact, I am a girl, not a boy. According to my dad; girls don't chew gum, boys can, and girls don't sit with their legs apart, not even when wearing trousers. Girls don't drink spirits, only small glasses of wine.

I mean come on! Was he born in the twenties? He is so sexist. If he only new what his little innocent girl had done in her short life. I can drink a bottle of whiskey on my own. I don't know any guy who can do that. I lost my virginity before puberty. He is so protective because I am a girl. Does he not realise I do not need protecting. I have done it all already. I have more life experience than him and I am only 17 years old. Has he not noticed this? He isn't the good role model he claims to be. Leaving your wife for a friend of hers is not something to look up to. He left us again and again and again before he finally decided to divorce my mum.

From the age of 8 years old I had my mother crying at my bedside telling me of the things he was doing with other women. I felt sick to know how weak she was. My grandfather was even more fucked up. How on earth does he expect me to think of him as a good role model and good parent? He never looked after me when I was little. No that is the women's job. Is it any wonder that I hate men? Is it any wonder that I refuse to be degraded because I am a woman? I will never marry a man like my father. I would gladly rather die, rather then be as weak as my mother was and put up with his shit. She should have taken him to court or beat him up years ago. He didn't even want to marry her. He never even loved her. It is men like my dad who give all men a bad name. Stuck in their ways and scared a woman can do things better than them. Is it any wonder that I am fucked up?!

We did art today. I have never done that in a hospital before. Everyone relaxed and mucked about for a while. I don't get on with many of the patients here. They are all a lot older than me. Still there is one guy here who is gay. He is nice. He is a day patient though so he leaves in the afternoon. Apart from him everyone else is dull and boring.

The staff here are okay. I have to have nurses sit with me at night because my doctor thinks I will hurt myself otherwise. Funny thing is that I have not cut since I came here. My psychiatrist is very nice. I call him Doc, or Dr. Mc Fab. It was a name that I started but other patients have picked it up. He has so many nicknames: Flip Flop, Big Mac, George Clooney's twin, Bugs Bunny, Mr. Fix It. The list goes on. He is the first psychiatrist who has made me laugh. He also seems to understand me. Maybe not all shrinks are dicks. He seems to know what he is talking about. All the patients here like him because he doesn't treat you like a patient. He doesn't look at you like the other doctors do. He actually seems interested when he asks you how you are feeling or if the meds are helping at all. He makes treatment bearable. At least there are some doctors in the world who can make a difference and who haven't forgotten why they wanted to do this job.

I kind of miss one of my last schools. Lucy, Hattie, Alice and Frankie were the group of girls I would hang around with. We were all so different. Like a huge pick a mix bag. I don't think that they new about how bad my self-harming was getting. They knew about it and I remember showing Alice once because she didn't believe me. Hattie had self-harmed too. She had once cut with a knife and needed stitches. Miss. Urquhart our housemistress had taken her to get stitches. Our housemistress was cool. I remember she always made me laugh. She had a great sense of humour and was really sweet. She always let me get away with little things that I shouldn't have done. She seemed to know just how do deal with me in the right way. We weren't allowed jewellery in that school, but I had eighteen piercings that I wanted to show off. Every day Miss. Urquhart would confiscate one or two bits from me. When I finally left after four years she gave me a huge bag, filled with earrings and bracelet's etc...that I had forgotten about.

I have always hated school. Teachers thought I was lazy and never pushed myself with my school work. The actual fact was that I had learning difficulties and would be at school from eight am to eight pm on most nights leading up to my GCSE'S and I also had school on Saturdays and had had extra tuition since I was five years old. I still got terrible grades and my dad would always yell at me for not trying even harder. At 16, and even now I don't think I could have tried harder than I did. My school reports were always bad and I was suspended for things like swearing at a teacher or being caught with a knife in my bag. I was a London kid at heart but had suddenly been put into these country schools and having to make a very quick switch from Kensington to Gloucestershire.

Hattie and I used to get drunk at each other's houses. We would down a bottle of whisky between us and sing loudly to cheesy S club 7 songs, which for some reason Hattie had purchased. In the mornings after blaming mysterious stains on the living room rug on her dog, Bob, we would go to school assembly still drunk. Over the school day we would sober up, only to go home and get drunk again. We never drank for fun but to pass out. We would sit the remainder of the night with our heads over buckets and running to the loo every five seconds to pee. Sometimes when we knew we couldn't make it up the stairs and down the hall we would use the kitchen sink. I will never forget the time

89

her mum discovered a poo in the fireplace. That Hattie also blamed on poor Bob. When we were at my house we would sit in a green house at the bottom of the garden that I used as an art studio. Even though it was November we would curl up on the floor with my brindle bulldog Lilly and almost freeze to death all night long on the concrete floor. We would share a big bottle of Red Bull and vodka that tasted like cough medicine and was just as thick and sweet. I would buy loads of them and smuggle them over from Switzerland. Hattie seemed to understand me most at that school. She was rebellious like me but had a rare charm that let her get away with it.

She came on holiday to Switzerland with me once; we were about fourteen at the time. We had gone to the pub to pick up hot guys. I had pulled two blokes under my sister's watchful eye. On the way home Hattie and I got into a fight. I ended up giving a blowjob to some desperate European bloke and Hattie had slapped me. Why, I never could remember. I think it was the only time in my life that she had been angry with me. The next day with hangovers we hit the slopes. Hattie managed the entire mountain on her bum, freezing to death in a Miss Selfridges jacket and stopping for fag breaks, which took thirty-five minutes because it was so hard to light up due to the wind. It seems like ages ago. A time before I went into treatment centres but I miss those years because they seem easier than now.

In school we learnt certain life skills like how to write a cheque and what jobs we would like to do. We talked about sex and drugs. They never taught us what to do if our friend was self harming even though at one point I had three in my year doing it. They never opened our eyes to mental illness or that statistically most of us would experience depression in our lives, one of us would kill ourselves and that some would have eating issues. They didn't tell us who to call if our parents abused us or that two of us will get raped.

The Other Patients: On my unit there was a mixture of patients who all had as big a mixture of ages. There was no one my age. There was no one under the age of twenty-nine. Most were in their early forties, or so they claimed. Some were doubtful. They were in there for several different things the majority being depression. I never got on very well with any of the patients but enough to be able to have a conversation. Over time there were a few I bonded with but I didn't stay in contact with any of them. One woman who I got to know well died soon after I left. She jumped in front of a bus.

I think that I am leaving soon. I am going to another hospital. I have actually been given a choice. I have chosen the one where my doctor works. Then I don't need to start over again with a new psychiatrist. I am scared though. I don't want to leave. This will be my fourth treatment in a row. I am starting to miss my friends from the outside. I haven't heard from my brother in months. He might call me tonight though. I don't know what I will say to him. I don't think he knows much about what has happened. I don't know how much my parents have told him.

I am leaving tomorrow. I don't want to. I hope they let me keep my mobile phone. I might have to hide it. I am going to the next hospital because I am an alcoholic, apparently….But I don't think I am. I do drink heavily though, but maybe I am not addicted. I want to cut but I won't. I don't want to disappoint the staff. I want to run away. I spoke to my brother the other day. It went well. I didn't know what to talk about so I let him do most of the talking. I think he was a bit nervous about what to say, but at least I know he cares. He kept doing jokes to make me laugh and his good Rik Mayal impressions really cheered me up.

Departure: I left with a potted orchid in hand. It was a gift from my mother. Half of it broke off as I had mistakenly slammed the taxi door on it. I looked up and caught a glimpse of my bedroom window. Its blue colour glass and grey blinds. A nurse sat with me on the other side of the car, to escort me to my next hospital. As the cab turned out of the parking lot and on to the busy road I felt sad. It was still in view but I missed it already. My comfort zone was gone.

I AM NOT YOUR DAUGHTER

Don't look at me with those eyes; they burn into the very core of my soul. Stop asking those questions, I have answers but you would not want to hear them. Stay away from my life because I hurt everyone that I am close to. Don't try and heal what you can't understand. I am not you. I am not like you. Not that daughter that you brought home with love. I am something strange, different and complicated. I have evolved into someone crazy. Don't make me feel guilty when there are too many other things on my mind. How can I tell you what I want for dinner when I can't even decide whether I should die or live?

How can I soothe your unhappiness when I am suffering so much inside? Take away your rules and discipline. They are not welcome in my cold world. Dress me up for school in a rich girl's uniform, and tell your friends of my impressive goals for the future. But do not pretend to be surprised when finding my body tomorrow. It will be cold and lying in the bed your daughter once used to sleep.

Go to therapy, and run and ask the teachers about how you could have missed this. How you could have not realised my pain. Just open your eyes and see. I am standing right here in front of you. Blood seeping through the jumper you gave me for Christmas last year. It used to be a pale baby blue. Have you honestly not seen the red blood stains on it? Is my hurting so well concealed? Or do you just choose to block it out. Turn away, shut the door. My pain does not have room for the two of you. It contains only me.

My View on the Place: I think it was a good place for me to be in. I went throughout my entire stay with out self-harming once. I was happy there and enjoyed the staff and other patients company. My family often visited and I was at home. I don't exactly know what the difference was between that hospital and many others but this one seemed to work for me. I would and have recommended it to several people as well as my psychiatrist who worked there. I felt the nurses were mother figures to many of the patients and this helped many of them, including me. It was a relaxed, quiet unit and I believe that that was just what I needed.

How It Affected Me: I know that my stay was a positive one. I didn't self-harm once during my stay there. I had built up trust with my psychiatrist and it was the first time I was starting to understand why I did the things I did in my life, and that that was o.k. My parents started to get an understanding of who I was and who I would always be. It was a good place to be when on the start of recovery.

SHE SCREAMS

She screams and walks in silence,
Her past a dream, her future a vision,
The sky above her flashes memories,
That all seem dark and grey,
But there's a beam of light among them,
Showing her there's hope,
She can't always see it, but seldom sheds a tear,
Her feelings are locked up,
Inside where they are safe,
A dreamer, a something,
Her mind not always there,
She doesn't know who she is,
Or which path to take,
She screams, not many hear,
Her soul finds a way to escape from,
The box that is her life,
"Who can help me?"
She asks…

No one answers,
Her world is silent.

THE DIFFICULT PATIENT

So sweet and innocent,
Like a child she sleeps,
A stuffed toy in hand,
Mouth parted on her frowning face.

Her skin bruised and scarred,
Purple circles and marks,
Black stitches on deep cuts,
Burned skin on her wrists.

Scared of the dark,
Needing love,
Not admitting she is an adult,
Wanting to stay a little girl.

Looking for a father figure,
Trying to understand,
Flirting with any man,
Linking love with pain.

Mood swings constant,
Can't make up her mind,
Making threats of suicide,
Screaming of love and hate.

Craving to be by herself,
Crying when she is alone,
Wanting help so desperately,
Pushing caregivers away.

Wanting so badly to die,
The next minute needing to live,
Hating any human with a dick,
But fucking everyone she can.

Making herself ugly,

By layers of fat and battle wounds,
Not knowing when she is dreaming,
Praying her world isn't real.

Filling the emptiness inside her,
Knowing she is not worth the doctors time,
Manipulating to get what she wants,
But in desperate agony hoping some one will care.

CROSS THE BORDERLINE

Reach out, touch the darkness,
Ignore those danger signs,
Give in to its seduction,
And cross the borderline.
Sink in ever deeper,
Get lost within the night,
Relax and bath in lakes of blood,
Let its insanity be your light.
Be calmed by its understanding,
In childish manner with your mind it will play,
There is no return ticket,
Inside its grasp you forever will stay.
Let it show you affection,
By filling your heart with rage,
You have become its puppet
And your life is now the stage.
Sink into the blackness,
Let its evil become your emotions
Burn skin and slice at flesh,
As a symbol of endless devotion,
Step over the edge, cross the border,
Feel the emptiness consume your life,
Indulge in fantasies about death,
It will urge you to pick up the knife.

NEW LABEL

I close my eyes hoping what,
I see is just a dream,
When I open them everything,

Is still as it seems,
Have I gone crazy?
Is this a psychotic episode?
I don't know who I am,
Perhaps I'll never know,
There was a time when I thought,
The label on my back was permanent,
Now I have been branded once again,
I can't run,
My feet are in cement,
But why would I try to run?
Everywhere I go,
My problems go with me,
I know what it's like not to hear,
I feel like I'm blind and cannot see,
I want to scream,
But have no voice,
This label is tattooed,
I have no choice,
Each label I get,
Is putting wait on my shoulders,
A chain round my neck,
I'm dragging round boulders,
Each of the doctors I meet,
Smiles and acts like their God,
They want me to have faith in them,
I used to but now I do not!

NOT THE SAME

Why am I so different?
How could I be this way?
I am not like normal people.

I am the star that does not twinkle,
I am the bruise on a wounded child,
I am the shark in a sea of patients,
And I won't recover at a fast rate.

I enjoy pain to an extreme,
I do not fear death but welcome it,
I can relate to the insane,

I am the missing piece in the puzzle of smiles.

I am the impatient look on social workers faces,
I am the doctor's hopeless sigh,
I am the teacher's angry frown,
I am a psychologist's nervous breakdown.

I am the girl screaming in restraints,
I am the girl buying razors,
I am accompanied by voices you can't hear,
I am the one who sees things you don't.

MY SHELL

My eyes reflect emotions I try and hide,
My body bottling my feelings inside,
My skin has scars, a story it tells,
This isn't me you're seeing,
This is just a shell.

You think I'm a strong woman handling this world,
You don't realise I'm just a frightened little girl,
You presume I'm getting better, that I'm well,
This isn't me you're seeing,
This is just a shell.

My smile is what I show you,
My happiness is so far from true,
My sanity seems to be flying, but in fact it fell,
This isn't me you're seeing,
This is just a shell.

To you I seem alive, but my mind says I'm dead,
To you I don't cry because my tears are red,
To you I act free but I'm trapped in a cell,
This isn't me you're seeing,
This is just a shell.

In your eyes my wounds are healing,
In your eyes I'm slowly feeling,
In your eyes you do not see my hell,
This is not me you're seeing,

This is just a shell.

WHY?

How could my life rise,
And bloom into hell?
Will I ever feel sunlight,
On my pale face?
Why is he filled,
With hopeless horror?
When through his eyes will,
I not be a disgrace,
Why must I walk the path,
Of life in the dark?
When will I not feel,
Dazed and confused?
When will I not be,
A frog among swans?
When will those who listen,
Look concerned and not amused?
Will I ever be loved so much,
It makes me hurt?
When will I stop cutting,
And freeing Scarlet streams?
When will I be happy,
In a place where I am free?
There is no place for me,
Except for in my dreams!

CHAPTER FOUR

London-2 Hospital.

May-June
17 years old

Arrival: The rooms were small and after having been sitting on my bed for half an hour I got sent downstairs to the cafeteria. I was met by staring eyes that scanned my appearance. Yes yet again I was wearing that snake print skirt. It had made a come back by then to the horror of many patients and my psychiatrist.

First Impression: A very small unit. It was claustrophobic. There were no self-harmers. Only detox patients. More tunnels. This is not where I belonged. It was too easy to escape. I could have run. I had the route planned out in my mind.

The Professionals: I had the same psychiatrist as I had had when in the first London hospital. I liked this because it didn't mean that I would have to build up trust again. I saw him regularly and could talk to him more and more about anything that bothered me. He seemed more relaxed in this hospital and joked around more with other patients. This made me more at ease to and it helped me to communicate to him what was worrying me. By this stage he was and still is used to me rambling on for ages about nothing very important. However just that alone helped in a strange way.

FEELING DEAD

Sometimes for no reason I feel dead. I feel numb, as if I'm floating. I never know when it will happen, or what triggers it, that's for the professionals to figure out. It is however horrible. I will some times walk down the street and wonder if people can see me. If I walk by someone I will jump in front of them to make sure they react. If they do, I know I am real, that I am a living person, that this fucked up life actually does belong to me. Other times I will have to cut. I absolutely must see my fat and muscle to believe I am alive. But mostly it is my blood. I need to see it to make sure it's there. I debate it in my mind or out loud. If there is blood there must be a heart to pump it. Then I must be alive, right?

To most people this sounds strang but then again most people are not like me. They go through life worrying about bills, their jobs, kids, and partners. They don't worry about whether that voice screaming in their ear can be heard by anyone else, or if that distorted shadow at the window whilst driving can be seen by anyone else. They don't need to worry that they are dead or if they are just dreaming.

Usually when I do a very deep cut it is when I think I am dreaming. Only when the bleeding will not stop do I suddenly realise I am awake. It is like when you are a young child and you are sleeping. You need the bathroom so you see yourself get up, walk out your room, into the bathroom, sit down and relieve yourself. It is only then that you wake up and find you are still in bed with a wet sheet... But you were so sure you got up. You were so sure you were not dreaming.

That's what its like for me. I think I am dreaming, so its o.k. to cut. Then when I have cut too deep and realised I am real, the consequences of rushing to the A and E come into play. It is however a good way to tell if a person is like me or not. Much like how any junkie can spot another one in a crowd. If I say a weird idea, or strange thought I am having to some one and they nod. I know they are like me. If they get freaked out, I know they are not.

It sounds weird and crazy. I am aware of that. I have seen too many people try and hide their shocked and confused faces, to know it is not normal. Only with another nut patient can you have a conversation like, "how are you feeling?
"Oh I'm good, how about you?"

"Well I am feeling a bit dead today," and know they fully understand what you mean.

The Regular Staff: Most of the nurses were great with few exceptions. There was one in particular who was very motherly and this seemed to help most patients especially me. She was more relaxed and kinder than the other staff. She let us misbehave more, but could definitely put her foot down when the time came. The other nurse's were fun too and showed us a more human side of the job. The therapists were all liked too. The atmosphere in groups was enjoyable compared to most.

The Other Patients: Most, well every patient on my unit was in there for drugs or alcohol addiction. Everyone seemed to gather into his or her own little groups of choice. The junkies hung around with the crack heads, methadone addicts and anyone else that took more serious drugs. They seemed to look down on people who took coke and those who smoked weed. The alcoholics stuck to themselves. They didn't like me, whoever I was, so the junkies took me into their group. For the most part the patients were moody and aggressive when coming off their drug of choice, but after that they were ok. Many had been in there several times before, and I was sure that in the future they would be back. A lot of patients walked out when they couldn't handle the program, and I rarely saw them again. One girl in particular who was only five years older than me seemed to bond with me fast. She was the only one who I stayed in contact with when I left. She is the only ex-junkie I have known to date that has made such a complete turn around of her life. She is my example of a view that if a program doesn't work then life will.

THE NIGHTS

The nights were usually quiet. Apart from someone coughing up mucus, or a junkie moaning, or the security guard snoring down at the front desk, it was silent. Empty. The chaos of rehab was temporarily numbed for just a few hours. No one seemed to be around. They were all behind closed doors scheming about how they could get the nurse to give them more Librium and Diazepam. They lay in their rooms, asleep pondering over their past, or feeling sorry for themselves, victims. I hated them for it. Esther and I refused to live like that. We were in our own world not theirs. 'Es' and I were not the same but we understood each other anyway.

It was on this night, like every other night that we sat together in the small kitchen. The bright neon lights that were fitted over the small table stung our eyes. The barred window was open a crack and the wandering bugs drawn in by the light would smack into the hot glass, fall flightless through the air and then buzz on the wood of the table. Once they had recovered they would simply fly up to the same light get knocked down again. It was as if they were mesmerised. It reminded me of Es and all the other addicts on the unit. No matter how badly they got hurt, or how many times they fell, they still carried on towards their drug, over and over again just like the bugs did with the light.

We looked odd together. There was Es with her short dark thick hair. Mine was long, blonde and very fine. She was tall with small breasts and had hardly any meat on her. I had large breasts, was short and chubby due to a year sitting around in hospitals yet we had so much in common. Neither of us understood the world we lived in. We couldn't relate to normal, happy people. We had both long ago decided to be patients for life. Both of us were in hospital but knew we wouldn't get better. We were what I call lifers. Patients who had lived the way we did so long that we had forgotten what normal life was. Es and I were the kind of patients that doctors didn't want to deal with because they knew that we were not going to be fixed straight away. It would take nothing short of a miracle to change who we were.

Shadows under our eyes from lack of sleep; we sipped our coffees and took long, desperate drags from our cigarettes. We never slept. Well I never slept. I could keep going for as long as four days without sleep. Sometimes we both could survive weeks with only three hours sleep a night. We didn't need it. Just sitting there in the quiet darkness was enough rest. Those few hours when we sat there, hair hanging down over our faces, my pashmina covering my slashed arms, her sleeves pulled up over her knuckles, was our break. It was the only rest we got in our hectic dysfunctional lives. The only time we had when the world just stopped spinning. When we could take a deep breath before the sun rose again and our depressing lives began.

Departure: As usual when I left I felt sad. Sad to leave the first psychiatrist I had ever trusted. Sad to leave the staff that had put up with me for so long. It was sad to leave the memories, and other patients. It felt like I was leaving my home.

My View on the Place: It didn't help me come to terms with my disorder. It didn't help me fit in with those like me. It was and still is a good place for addicts to get on the right road of life. I am grateful that I went there but it was more fun than anything else. Like a break from the everyday stresses people cope with. However I would not want to go there for treatment of any sort again. I would recommend it for addicts I knew who wanted good treatment but couldn't afford some of the more expensive hospitals.

LAUNDRY

We messed about a lot. Like children we would come up with little naughty plans that got us into trouble. We were making up for the years in our childhood when we didn't get to play. We had had to grow up fast and new we were taking back the years we had lost. Es had grown into a junkie. She had a degree in heroin and had all the qualifications of other drugs. I had chosen a medical career and was now a self-harmer specialising in razors and cutting. *I had passed most exams in mental health and was now a Borderline.*

Es got bored easily but I liked a challenge. Instead of university I had chosen hospitals and treatment centres. I was a difficult patient but I thought that that was my job. On one of our cheeky occasions when we both needed our lives on the unit spicing up, we decided to go to the laundry room. The machines were old and rusty. Piles of clothes were in baskets, covered in vomit and blood. I saw one large basket that had wheels on it. Before I had said anything Es had read my mind. Jumping in she waited for me to push her. I did. It was as if she was a massive baby in an oversized buggy. Cries of laughter and screams of excitement came from her mouth. I had never heard her so happy before. I ran down the corridors almost sending her flying as I turned the corners.

After about five minutes we both started noticing the smell. We couldn't figure out what it was or where it was coming from. Some new drunk must have come into the ward. The stench of him was unbearable. Es suddenly stopped laughing. She complained that her tight jeans felt wet. Before she could say anything else she jumped out of the basket. She had been sitting in urine soaked sheets without realising. I didn't want to know what else might be on them. We ran screaming to our separate rooms to wash. It was a time that I will never forget. A typical example of how our fun experiences in life end terribly. However, without them I could never have survived my life without the ability to laugh about every situation whether good or bad. To be able to share that with someone is even more special.

How It Affected Me: It gave me a good friend that I have shared so much with and for that I am grateful. It helped me build a trusting and fun relationship with my psychiatrist that I still have today. It gave me social skills and memories for a lifetime. It made me aware of the fact that I am not an alcoholic though doctors in the past have claimed I was. It has made me realise that someone from a different lifestyle and background can still totally connect with what I am feeling.

DOC

I am like you, but tainted. My frown is just a smile turned upside down. My disorder is like your happiness but is just turned inside out. My mind is the same as yours but back to front. My life is like a piece of paper, lying crumpled on the floor. Your memories held in your heart, mine are put away, sealed in a box, in a dark place that no one will ever find. You hear a small voice reminding you to do something. I hear a morbid collection of voices reminding me to kill my self. But we are still the same, just....not.

Unfold me. Take me gently in your hands and with delicate movements straighten me out. Make me smooth. Make me normal. With a thick brush paint a bright red smile across my face so that at least on the outside I look happy. Give me a list of believable lies that I can tell people when they ask me where I have been all this time. Let them not know the truth. Let their doubt in me guide them away from the real places I have been. The hospitals, the treatment centres, the rehabs, the nut houses that they only know from magazine gossip columns and movies. Let them not know that people like me exist in their bubble wrapped world. Let their parents not know that I a crazy woman live on their street. Across from their white picket fenced doll houses.

Please! Mould me like clay in your hands until I resemble a sane person. Ramble on in our sessions about anything, at least then for a few minutes I can stop my thoughts from spinning. Can you fix me? With paper and glue cover up my scars so the world cannot see how I hurt myself. Take nails and a hammer and patch up the wholes in my mind that leak out these crazy thoughts. Take down from the shelf that huge medical book. Read to me about my disorder so I know it is real. Tell me statistics and percentages of those who have it also, so I know I am not alone. Give me promises, even if fake, about how I will survive this hell. How I will be alive this time next year. How you do, even though it is a job, care.

See past my childish face, my frown and eyes that show no fear, and see. See that I have no hope. That I am telling you lies. How I am desperate for something to get me through this chaos. Do not believe me when I say that I am feeling better. Use your knowledge to know that I am manipulating the truth and that inside I want to die. Stop writing notes. Instead look over your glasses and realise that tonight I am going to die. Please stop me before it is too late, before another Borderline dies. Read up on all the suicidal signs in patients and like a super hero stop me from ending my life. Fix me.

DON'T RELEASE ME

Don't ever release me from your grasp. Don't send me into a world non-understanding. Don't fill in the form that claims I have recovered and with pills in hand show me to the door.

I need your protection. I need your rules and structured timetable. I need your discipline. I need your punishment. I need it more than life.

I forever want your love, no matter how fake. I want your understanding, even if it is a job. I want you here with me, even if you are paid to be. I want to know you understand, even if a textbook shows you how.

I do not fit into that shiny life where the sun makes my eyes sting. I do not know how to blend with all those smiling faces. I do not know how to talk with laughter. I do not know normality in any sense. I do not know anything but this.

106

Keep me inside and away from them. Keep me with others like me. Keep me on my pills that calm. Keep me in groups where I can scream freely. Keep me alive. Keep me entertained. Keep me protected from the judging of those that are sane. Keep me from those that only know, "happiness."

Hold me in your padded arms. Hold me in your silver buckles and straps. Hold me contained within these walls. Hold me from myself. Hold me from the outside world, the one I have never been able to live in.

Feed me your knowledge of who I am. Feed me your patience. Feed me words of wisdom, which I cling to. Feed me your concerns of my arms. Feed me your anger when I misbehave. Feed me your big sad eyes when you learn how sick my mind is. Feed me news of the outside world that I have no use for. Feed me your wish for me to get better.

Don't take my only chance. Don't push me away when money runs out. Don't throw me to the wolves. Don't ruin my glimpse of hope by shutting me into the darkness. Don't release me. Don't ever unlock heavy security doors. Don't tell me to pack my bags and say my goodbyes. Don't have hope for me. Don't talk of other patients getting better, making me green in envy.

I am what I am. I need this place. I cannot survive out there. I will not put down the razor once free. I do not need a normal life. I do not need to be given a new chance at my fucked up life. I do not need a change of environment. I will just kill myself.

I need to be here. This is my sanity. This is my chance, my only life. This is what I need. This is all I want to know. This is what I crave for. This is who I am. This is who I will always be.

So don't release me. Do not talk of other patients who cut deeper than me, I only get jealous of the attention you are giving them. So don't focus on them when I need you more. Don't make me beg. Don't make me threaten suicide. Don't make me slice my arms to stay. Don't trust me on my own with all these pills. Don't trust me and my manipulating smile. Don't listen to me if I say I am happy, or I want to get well. Don't believe me when I say I am better.

AFFAIR

How could you do this?
You told me that you care,
About our relationship,
I know about your affair,
You claim I'm imagining things,
That you're not fooling around,
Yet you sneak out late at night,
Trying not to make a sound,
I catch you on the phone,
Trying to get her on the line,
She has been in our house,
In our bed you've had her,
I'm not that dumb or blind,
In your sleep you call out her name,
I knew she would be back,
You are leaving me for her,
This woman, this drug, called smack.

MY BODY

My body is not a temple,
And not a sacred place,
My arms are slashed from sadness,
My mind has gone to waste,
My eyes are dark and hollow,
And my hair goes un-brushed,
I am not used for beauty,
But instead for lust,
My nails go neglected,
And my lips are bitten raw,
Grazes mark my cheekbone,
As though I've been to war,

My right leg has a limp,
There are blisters on my feet,
I'm only seen at night,
Shifting from street to street,
My clothes are all worn out,
My shoes are just the same
Often my make up is smudged,
Not from tears but rain,
My body is not a temple,
And not a sacred place,
My arms are slashed from sadness,
My mind has gone to waste.

FIRST CUT

Why did you break the razor?
Do you remember that time?
Wasn't scratching enough for you,
Didn't you read the signs?
When you saw the blood,
And you felt such great relief,
That's when you should have known,
It was too good to believe,
You wondered how you could feel so great,
You wondered if it was wrong,
How could you think of consequences?
When you wanted this for so long.

HIS LIQUID GREEN, HIS METHADONE.

His liquid green,
His body slumped,
His eyes pinned,
All is lost.
Sugar to better the taste,
His words left unsaid,
His dream state begins,
All at such a cost.
His dark memories forgotten,
Surrounded by warmth,
So easy to drink,

He needed to pretend.
His heart rate not right,
Thick and sticky sweat,
Flashing lights and shouting,
The screaming of the siren.
His clothes cut off,
Induced vomiting,
Drips hooked up,
His body twitching; violent.
No more liquid green,
No more comforting warmth,
Now dream state does not end,
Now his world is silent.

YES, NO, MAYBE

I love you, no I don't,
Stop walking away!
I need you, but I'm independent,
Don't listen to what I say!
Why are you ignoring me?
You're my lover and my friend!
I'll stay with you forever,
This relationship must end!
I need you to be here for me,
I want to be alone!
Get out of my life,
Don't leave me on my own!
I hate you….sometimes,
I'm not messed up in the head!
I'll change because I love you,
But I just wish you were dead!

SWEET PILLS.

In packages and bottles,
Contain my lovely pills,
I line them up in a row,
And laugh at the thrill.
Green and white capsules,
Shiny round and oval bright,
Each one so enticing,

So quick to dissolve my fright.
Baby blues and palest pink,
Simple and easy to swallow,
So small and delicate,
Yet powerful enough to fill the hollow.
As I take one after the other,
And an infinity of time goes by,
I realise no one knows I'm here,
Trying not to cry.
No doctor new I was suicidal,
I wore my mask so well,
Doubt was all I got,
When I explained my hell.
I start getting drowsy,
And my breath starts to die,
That I have the guts to do this,
No one can deny.
I feel my heart pound slower,
My vision starts going blind,
I try and reach for the phone,
I've now changed my mind.
I don't want to die yet, ust wanted to end the pain,
I'm all alone down here,
My sweet pills, my only friends.

CHAPTER FIVE

Arizona-Treatment Centre.

June-July
17 years old

Arrival: I arrived in the car park in high flip-flops and was taken to the nursing station. They looked very worried when they saw my scars, and kept badgering me about when it was that I last cut. I was introduced to my peers on the adolescent unit and again I got the staring. I was told that I couldn't smoke. I was furious. I was not told this in England. I didn't care about anything except my cigarettes. I needed my nicotine to get me through this.

18/05/01
Well I've arrived at last! When I went through security at the airport, they ripped apart my bags, and searched every inch of them. I hate it when they do that! Then they just cram it in! They then fired questions at me, asking where I was going. I was pissed off as I was flying with my American passport. When I told them I was going to a treatment centre, they were suddenly really nice, and thanked me for choosing their country.

Then I was stuck in a car (which was fucking boiling,) for ages. The staff member who had picked me up kept rambling on about how brilliant the place was. I reminded her that I had paid already, and that she didn't need to convince me. That and the fact that it wasn't exactly my choice to go there, but was passed on. This will be my fourth treatment centre in a row. I haven't even had one day of freedom, before coming here. I can't figure out what's wrong with me. I'm not a sociopath. I can't be that hard to handle. Still at least it's not a nut house.

When we finally arrived, I almost collapsed as a heat wave attacked me. It was so funny. Every one could tell I was from England. I was the only one complaining about the heat. While I was in flip-flops, t-shirt and skirt, others were in jeans and jumpers. At least they don't have restraints here. The only thing that's worrying me is that if I do just the tiniest cut, I get thrown out, apparently. They are a lot stricter here than in London. They can't possibly expect me to stop just like that. It's my life support. I wish they could give me a self-harm.

Doc said they are good here. I think it's going to be a while before I see his point. The girls here seem really different. Not any one of them hears voices. None of them see hallucinations. I'm really hungry but can't eat anything because of my tongue stud. It's really swollen and has started to hurt a bit.

First Impressions: It is hot. It is boiling. It looks like a desert. No I am not mistaken, it is a desert. It looks more like a holiday resort than a treatment centre. This can't be the place; they have sent me on holiday! There are more cactuses than there are patients. Cactuses bloody everywhere, cactuses and sand…Cactuses, sand, the sun and one hell of a pissed off girl from England.

19/05/01
Today I feel really good about myself. I actually don't have any urges to cut. I have started to open up in-group a little, which is a good improvement for me. I feel as though I'm shining. Then again that could be the sunburn on my face. Damn this pale skin! In-group this afternoon, a girl started speaking about how her mom always threatened to leave, when she was little. Mom used to do that when I was really young. I barely remember it, but it happened. I hate it when memories come flooding back like that. It makes me wonder, just how much stuff I don't remember, or how much I have chosen to forget. Put to the back of my mind, to deal with another day.

All the girls here, well some of them; about seven, are really into Wicca (witch craft.) the staff told them I heard voices and now they think I'm some powerful

113

Goddess. It's so ridiculous. Maybe the kids are more fucked up than I thought. That or they have watched the craft too many times. There's a really cool girl here called Dana. She actually thinks that she is a vampire. I mean seriously, and then she wonders why she is here. She is so funny though. There is a Tec here called Chris. He has a tongue piercing and is going to help me clean it. It's still fairly swollen.

20/05/01

I am really pissed off! I fucking hate myself. All they were talking about in group today was how mental hospitals weren't bad and that only really disturbed people went there. They don't have a fucking clue. If they had been to one, and been molested by a staff member and patients they wouldn't say that. Then they were all complaining, and saying that this place was like a jail. It really makes me mad, I wish they were all locked up and gang raped! I feel like I want to kill myself again. I hate feeling like this, it's horrifying. Maybe I should grab a kitchen knife and slash my wrists and then kill all the patients and doctors here. My hallucinations are back.

My meds are being upped again, they still don't work. I know it takes time, but I wish they would be immediate. I might cheek them tonight and then snort them. That way I can get some sleep.

22/05/01

I did it and feel awful. It was in the shower with a pair of scissors. There was blood everywhere. I went out and told a Tec. I don't know why I did but they would have found out anyway. I had to then sleep on the couch in the nursing station, because they were out of beds, and they wanted to keep an eye on me. This really dumb nurse called Tab refused to dress it so I got lots of dirt and Dylan's hair in it. It's now really infected and they spent ages trying to pull the dirt out. It hurt like fuck. I'm now on a stupid one-to-one, with the coolest 24-hour nurse ever. I have been running round all day keeping her on her toes. She is the only one who listens to me.

I hate it here. They say they are going to send me to a place in Chicago but I don't want to go. Every time I get put somewhere I get passed on to another place. It sucks. I want to go back to the London.

23/05/01
Today I feel like shit. All my bandages keep falling off. The nurses can't even dress it properly. They won't let me do it. They won't let me go to groups either because of my anger. They say I'm too aggressive, and that I'm scaring some patients. My voices are really bad today too.

I'm so bored. I have spent the whole day talking to my 24-hour nurse, as I can't do anything else. She is actually really cool. I call her shadow, because that is what she is. She follows me everywhere I go. She seems to really care. She showed me how to make these beaded bracelets. I really admire her for coming here all the time, but still having a smile on her face. When I was allowed to go to the cafeteria at lunch all the patients starred at me. I hate that. They think I'm just some crazy girl who's going soon. My dad faxed me that the place I am going to is a hospital. If it's a nut ward I am going to really flip out. Next time I cut myself I am not going to tell anyone. The staff always say I should trust them. I don't, and never will again.
I feel like I'm letting everyone down. I always do.

26/05/01

Today I woke up feeling sad. I don't know why, there is no reason. The morning went o.k. It's Saturday so the staff are a bit more relaxed. I had bad period pains and it took me forever to get the nurses to let me have a pain killer. We had a very long and very boring group today. Doc called half way through, thank God, so I missed a lot of it. I was almost falling asleep listening to this girl ramble on about giving her little sister coke. He cheered me up though. It's such a relief to hear an English accent again.

This afternoon, I spoke to my mom. The whole day was fairly boring, and then finally some action happened. Mona and this girl called Anya locked themselves in their room. They used mattresses to block the door. The cops are being called, better than the restraint men. Every one is at an AA meeting in Tucson, except Dana and me. We have just been told to grab our blankets, a pillow, and go to the mobile, where we have groups, quickly.

We are now watching a lame video. The cops are here and there is so much commotion. I can't believe I am missing this. It's so exciting. I love pissing off the cops! On the way to the mobile we passed them. Dana and I started waving our arms around and trying to look really crazy, they tried to look really calm, and butch. Pity they weren't cute though.

The Professionals: My psychiatrist was completely unaware of what my disorder was and how to treat me. Compared to my doctor in England I would say that she needed to read a lot of books and re-take a few exams. I didn't like her mood swings. One day she was understanding and the next day she wouldn't have a care in the world about me or other patients. I felt uncomfortable around her and never felt at ease in her sessions. I didn't have a therapist in this hospital but I felt I really needed one. I wanted that private session. I wanted that one to one relationship with some one who could give me their full attention.

27/05/01

Mona has gone. She got discharged yesterday. They acted as if it was world war three. She is still coming back for family week though. She always makes me laugh; I'm going to miss her. She is such a slut. She has this thick red-brown hair, and bright green eyes, and looks like a war time French prostitute. I'm really scared. I have to work on my time line. I am presenting it to the group tomorrow. I'm worried of what every one will think of me afterwards.

28/05/01

The presentation went really well. They were really supportive and didn't flip out at all. I thought the doctors wouldn't believe me like in England, but they were cool about it all. I have been put on this weird medication that makes me feel really weird. It's for my stomach. The doctor said it had an abrasion in the wall due to drinking too much. I don't believe him. It must be because of something else.

29/05/01

Today has been a great day. I haven't had any voices at all. The meds aren't really working though. They upped them again. I had a great chat with my mum this afternoon.

This evening though something weird happened. There is this guy on the adult unit. He is a real dick and always smokes right in front of us, because he knows we aren't allowed to. So he was doing this when he left from the cafeteria, and we were all really pissed off. Then the funniest thing happened. He walked into a cactus. I mean that's the kind of thing you see in a movie. It was hysterical. I mean who actually walks into a cactus? It wasn't a little one either; it was one of those great big ones that are in western films. He was up in the nursing station for ages while the nurses tried their best to pull out all the spikes. A few hours later he emerged covered in a smelly cream. He looked ridiculous. That made my day.

30/05/01

I'm so stupid! Last night I was craving a fag really badly. I stormed out of the ward and kept harassing patients in the adult ward to give me some. I failed. Then I ran into the nurse's station and was yelling my head off at them for no reason at all, that I could think of. I don't know why I did it. I then started walking down the drive with about four staff running after me. After ages where I was holding a sharp stick to my throat in the middle of the road, they called the cops and I went back to the unit. They kept threatening to section me. I hate that. Shadow and I spent hours laughing about it. I now have a stomach ache. It was so funny. What was I honestly going to do with a stick?! It was more like a twig. My roommate Jenna was really cool. We pushed our beds together and stayed up the whole night making jokes about the doctors.

The Regular Staff: most of the staff there were good. I had a nurse who went everywhere with me. She helped teach me to talk through my problems and try asking for help, even though she wasn't asked to. The mental health technicians were all fairly young. They wore what they wanted and had a less superior image than most would. They didn't talk to us about their experiences or let us talk to them when we needed to. They wanted to give us a strict structured day to day plan of how to spend our time. They were fun though and would often join us, by choice, during game time.

06/06/01

Today was really cool. Most of the groups were good and my psychiatrist wasn't being a total bitch for once. Then this evening most patients went to AA. Me, Dana, Lilly and Brittany were left. Shadow gave us a video recorder and we messed about for hours with it. We made a short film about ourselves and even shadow joined in. She was playing a nurse doing checks and I was running around all psychotic. Dana was trying to escape through an open gate, Lilly was possessed by something and Brittany was being a bimbo all evening.

Like walking into trees and tripping over everything. It was hysterical. We got so into it that two hours later we realised a big group of adults had gathered to watch us. They had seen it all and started cheering. It was embarrassing. When the others came back we were yelled at though and even though shadow protested they took the camcorder and erased all our funny sketches.

YOU LIE

I flipped out today. My shrink told me to tell her what was bothering me. I told her that I thought my voices were real and there was no possibility that they are just in my mind. Then she gave me the look. The one every patient like me knows. The one that tells you to shut up, you have said something wrong, something bad. She looked and she looked. She scribbled in her note pad, and then fired questions at me. I answered no to all of them. I wasn't in love with an alien, I didn't think the devil was in me, I didn't think she was after me, I didn't think my food was being poisoned.

Every patient knows, when you get that look, you lie. You lie as if your life was on the line. You smile and you laugh and you act like a normal teen. You act as if it was a joke, or a thought you were not serious about. You know that if the shrink sees through you, you'll be put back into psychiatric. I left smiling. I left calm. But deep inside I know, I still think they are real.

07/06/01
Well today has been eventful. We were allowed to go to the pool and we were all craving anything fun. A girl called Jessie had found some fags by the side and had given them to me. I very obviously put them in a pencil case. Then the staff announced that we were all going to be searched. Jessie and I confessed and were taken to the nursing station. We got strip searched even after we gave them up. It's so dumb, it's not like we are going to shove fags inside our pussies.

119

Then we got yelled at for flirting with the adults. They took the whole thing so seriously. When we got back they told us the fags had been mixed with other shit. I was so pissed off. If we had known that we would have never given them away.

The Other Patients: I was among the oldest of the patients. Most of them were under seventeen and in the adolescent unit there were only girls. This made the group very bitchy. There was less aggression in the groups but a lot more manipulation between us. Most of them suffered from depression and minor eating disorders. Some had self-harmed in their past but didn't have an issue with it anymore. One girl was in there for cocaine abuse, two were in there for crystal meth. Most of the patients just seemed lost. Few of them liked me. I was the one who always got more attention due to my constant fake suicide threats and self-harm. I took staff time away from them and they resented this. In general they thought I was crazy. The ones that didn't hate me idolised me because they thought crazy was cool. I am not currently in contact with any of my peers from my unit.

08/06/01

This morning was really shit. It has been really hard not to cut. I did though and I feel guilty. I didn't tell anyone, they just get angry. They don't know what its like. It's not as if I have a choice.

I feel like I am disappointing everyone. The staff say I'm getting better. If only they knew, that behind my forced smile I have a cut so deep that I've gone through the fat and almost can see the veins. If they did they would just stitch it up. I don't like stitches. They hurt. It's funny that a self-harmer can be scared of a little needle and thread but not a carving knife. Actually I have met self harmers that are babies when it comes to any other pain, I'm one of them.

This afternoon, my toilet broke down. My shadow was sitting on the seat, watching me shower and then suddenly water came flooding everywhere. It was hysterical. She managed to fix it though. It made me laugh.

10/06/02
I'm sitting in the nursing station again. I seem to spend more time in here than in groups. I had to spend another night on the couch in the waiting room. It is so unpleasant to wake up with some very serious looking patients, and scared parents staring down on you.

I am listening to KFMA rock station de Tucson. I've got bandages all up my arms, I look like a mummy. I've been scratching at them like mad. I couldn't find anything sharp so I used my nails to rip off the skin that insists on healing my arm. The pain is different from cutting. It burns. It burns bad. I feel as if I really am turning crazy. Maybe I am.

The nurse here, Tab, has been giving me pills every four hours. They have a strong calming effect. Not like when you are high, but when you are so tired it's hard to move. All my actions now take more effort. I feel like I'm falling. My body is heavy, but I am still aware of everything around me. Then as soon as I have more energy they give me another. They say I'm too aggressive to go to groups. They say I might hurt some one. They don't understand my world. They are observers. Asking me how I feel every half hour. I wonder if this is some new drug that they have never tried before.

Time leaves me a lot. I will suddenly be aware of the time but not how I spent it. I am used to that, but now I am panicking. Is it the pills or me? I keep asking my shadow what I have done. She says I have been daydreaming for a long time. I'm glad she does not know about disassociation yet. I don't want her to become one of them. I like that she doesn't look at me the way they do. The way every one does when they know who I am, what I am.

121

I feel like I literally can't stop cutting. It's the only thing I am in control of. My shadow says it's the only thing I can't control. There is one nurse here who keeps threatening to section me. She laughs when she says it. Do doctors know what that means? Do they know the fear they create in me when they do that? It's a joke to them. I think they are sick.

My psychiatrist here is weird. Then again most are. I don't think they are human. They are born to do what they do. She told me perhaps I should get better. Funny, I never actually considered that. She acts like it's my choice to stay sick. As if it were a dream of mine to be like this forever. I must admit, there is a comfort in not being normal. But if she thinks that I don't want to get better, then she doesn't understand a thing. It's not like I pop a pill and hey presto I'm happy. Voices gone... violence gone... cutting gone... She says that I am more normal than I think and that I think that I am crazy when I am not. I am a borderline but that doesn't mean I have lost my mind. I am not capable of killing someone, or living in a made up world etc... I think she is crazier than me.

12/06/01
I walked off the premises again. I was screaming my lungs out. I don't know why. For some reason I couldn't stop rocking. They fed me lots of pills. I slept all day. Its 7:35pm now and at 8:00pm I am allowed to go to Dana's goodbye group, if I am good until then. She is leaving tomorrow very early, to go back to Oklahoma. It's no wonder she thinks she is a vampire if she grew up there.

I just spoke to a therapist in Chicago she seemed a total bitch. I think I will be leaving soon. They won't tell me when my discharge date is. I hope its tomorrow.

Departure: I was not very sad when I left. I didn't mind the patients but I was tired of the whole program. There were only a few girls I got on with but they had left and now I was ready to go. I had to board a plane with an

122

escort. I was too busy worrying about the new place that I was going to rather than leaving this one. I was praying they had air conditioning at the next hospital. I wasn't used to this heat.

13/06/01
I can't believe this. They say I am going to be here till Friday. I'm so confused, I didn't want to leave at first but now I do. I'm so bored without Dana. My shadow is trying to entertain me with stories of her past. She is so funny. She is hooked on anything Disney.

My hallucinations are back. They keep tapping on the window and scaring me. My shadow is telling me not to look, but it's hard. They are writing in blood on the glass. They want me to kill someone. Usually when I write like this they go away. It isn't working. I don't want them to come in. I hate them so much. I can't tell the staff because then they flip out and stuff me with pills. Maybe I should kill them. If I kill myself they will go away. But will I be dead then to? Maybe I will wake up. Maybe this is just a dream. I need to cut to make sure. Maybe this is not a real world. If I die I will wake up in the other world where my body is. Maybe this is all made up. Maybe my voices are not real. Am I imagining them when I get into this kind of state?

My shrink says I can have psychotic episodes. Is this one? The fact that I am dreaming isn't psychotic, is it? I don't understand. They never tell me everything. They only tell me small chunks of things. I don't understand life, if this is what it is. I only know what I know. My world, my blood, my voices. If they don't tell me what is normal how can I know how to get better.

When I am thirty I am going to kill myself. Then we will see who is right or wrong. Then I will either die, or wake up from this dream. But for now I will act normal. It is so easy to fool staff sometimes. If I twitch when I hear my voices, or jump when my hallucinations startle me, I laugh. I blame it on a spider or an itch. I have to pretend. I don't want to be locked up. The staff in nut houses can hurt you and get away with it. Does my shrink know that? Does she know how many sick people work there? That no-one believes what you say? Maybe I should be locked up. I could never live in the normal world.

My View on the Place: I think it is a very good treatment centre and it has a very good program for helping people with various problems. If I had the choice I would go back there in the future if I needed to and I have told several people in need of help about it. I feel that if I hadn't left it wouldn't have helped me, but that is because I didn't want to be helped. If I had gone in with a different attitude I believe it could have really done me some good.

How It Affected Me: It gave me a lot of self confidence. I did tasks there I thought I was too stupid to possibly ever be able to do. It gave me a lot of time to reflect on the life I once wanted to end. It gave me space from my parents, which now looking back, I think was good for me. It helped me grow as a person. It allowed to me act like a child again in a safe environment.

MY BADGES

When you are so far away from reality, death does not scare you. You feel such great relief to see that blood run down your arm. To know you're awake and not just dreaming. To know that if you were to peel back the layers of your skin, you won't be hollow inside. I search for that void. The one doctor's say patients like me have. They must be wrong, for I find only veins and muscle. Yet I still feel it hiding a big, dark, empty hole.

I was shit at school. I bet I could pass Biology now. I know where the bulging arteries lie, and the threatening blue lines that urge you to press down on them. That dare you to go deeper every time. I wish I were one of those people who turned crazy at age 20. But I always remember being like this. That little girl lost,

124

permanently. That little girl lost who is playing with her blood on the stained floor; who was purposely misbehaving because there was pleasure too in punishment and being too scared of crying for the fear of never stopping. Some girls join the Brownies or the Girl Scouts. They get patches for their courage. I go to treatment centres and psych wards…But I too get badges. My scars are badges and each one I earned. They do not get put in a draw and forgotten. They are engraved. Some are for years, others for life. They tell my story. They are like a diary written in blood on skin.

CREATURE OF THE NIGHT

I am a creature of the night,
A sliding shadow of darkness,
Dodging normal living at every chance,
My memories faded like the moonlight I walk in,
Making my way down the cracked pathway to hell,
My movement simple,
My eyes focussed on my destination,
As I pass those like me,
I turn from their stares,
Fearing they will look into my soul,
And see my secrets,
Then it begins,
The shameful sin with the devil,
Sucking out every piece of goodness,
In me I have left,
The red stream of emotions,
Runs from my veins,
That are gasping for life,
It ends,
And I close the gate to the memory in my mind,
And throw its key away,
Forever.

PICTURE PERFECT

A picture hangs upon the wall,
I used to not care at all,

An ugly thing to which I could not relate,
Its dark frame I did hate.

After time I grew used to it's sight,
And though I tried with all my might,
I could not get it out of my head,
So I lay there pondering in my bed.

It represented something I did not know,
A place of peace with happiness sowed,
The children in it smiled with glee,
But they did not seem to smile at me.

It tormented me with its view,
It was not my home; and that I knew
Deep inside I craved that place,
Where I too could have a smiling face.

TOO LATE

You realised that cutting,
Was better than scratching,
Instead of the burning from your nails,
The cool razors edge was relaxing.
There were soon scars on your arms,
You did well to cover them up,
Years later, now you've had enough?
Whether you are sane, or crazy,
Is your on going debate, You can't stop cutting now…
It is far too late.

THE CURSE

The curse it is set in blood, not stone,
And it will be made in the light of the moon,
The will for them all to die, a horrid way,
Their bodies melting and sinking under the earth,
The maggots they feast, no flesh is to waste,
And the bleeding skin crumples and shrinks,
The sorrow filled eyes that plead and beg,
Their soul's barley escaping the hands of hell,
Too late to repent, too late to say sorry,

126

My will has been made,
There's no turning back,
For their mistakes, every one will know,
That to mess with me, even the devils won't do,
So dare if you must,
But in the end you will pay like the rest.

STRAWBERRY KISSES

A strawberry kiss,
Make it sting,
Make it burn,
A strawberry kiss,
Is what I've earned.

A strawberry kiss,
Make it feel,
Make it real,
A strawberry kiss,
That will never heal.

A strawberry kiss,
My only friend,
No need to pretend,
A strawberry kiss,
Let this be the end.

A strawberry kiss,
Make me know pain,
Make me play the game,
A strawberry kiss, I need it again.

A strawberry kiss,
Make me see harm,
Make me the alarm,
A strawberry kiss,
Take me to the funny farm.
A strawberry kiss,
Is what I yearn,
I can never learn,
A strawberry kiss,
Make sure I never return.

DON'T TRY AND STOP ME

I've made up my mind,
I'll do it with a knife,
Don't try and stop me,
To end my bitter life.

I've made up my mind,
To you I will lie,
Don't try and stop me,
I just want to die.

I've made up my mind,
I'm in so much fear,
Don't try and stop me,
It's becoming so clear.

I've made up my mind,
I can't go on,
Don't try and stop me,
I've wanted this for so long.

I've made up my mind,
I want to bleed,
Don't try and stop me,
This I do need.

I've made up my mind,
But I can't stop the blood,
Don't try and stop me,
It's becoming a flood.

I've made up my mind,
I have said my goodbyes,
Don't try and stop me,
Let me close my eyes.

I've made up my mind,
I have planted the seed,
Don't try and stop me,
You won't succeed.

CHAPTER SIX

Chicago-1 Treatment Centre.

July-August
17 years old

Arrival: It looked welcoming from the outside. Inside there were more tunnels. I felt sick and heavy as I went through the heavy, glass locked doors. I knew they only meant one thing. I didn't like those doors. They represented no escape. It meant they contained patients who wanted to escape. I knew there would be restraint rooms. I knew the windows would not open all the way. I knew I would be eating with plastic forks. There wouldn't be any knives. My relaxed and tired body grew more and more tense. I became defensive. Weeks of hard work went out the window and I resorted to acting like a frightened little child, as I clutched a teddy in my hand. I didn't want to deal with this all over again. My life is a circle of dysfunction and chaos. I felt I had lived so many lives within the time period of my age.

17/06/01
Well I'm here now at the program. It's not as bad as I thought it would be. It's a locked unit though, in a big hospital. I never thought Chicago would look like this for some reason.

I'm worried though. I am not going to want to talk about some things. It's kind of strange that everyone here is a cutter. We had a group today and two women were saying how they never react the way most do in a situation. One woman said her friend had died in a car crash, and that instead of crying she cut, and instead of feeling sorry for the person, she envied her. It's weird, I have never realised that maybe there are people like me. Everything she was saying I could relate to. Instead of telling her she was not normal, the staff said in self harmer's it is very common.

I feel very relieved that here I can talk about my voices and not be looked at strangely. The patients here seem to understand in some way or another. I feel a little more normal. I can call people back home whenever I want, which is cool. They never let you do that in Arizona.

To get here was an ordeal. I had to fly with a nurse, who kept giving me medication, in case I ran. I felt completely numbed out. I guess people could tell what was happening because at the airport everyone kept starring at us, and asking my nurse questions about me. I slept most the way.

When I arrived it was late and I got introduced to a young guy called Calvin. He was going to be my therapist. All the other patients have a woman. I'm his only patient. He looks too young to know how to handle me. Then again, they say all the staff here have done some sort of self harm. That's kind of cool. I think it makes them understand more. It was never like that in England. I can't exactly picture Mc Phillips slicing up his arms every night.

First Impression: When I first arrived I was scared. I was so used to moving from place to place. I put up a defence immediately. I did not smile. I would not let them control me, or get inside my head. It was like wearing an invisible coat of armour. One that got heavier and heavier and harder to wear after some time. I couldn't wait to take it off and open up.

18/06/01
I have a roommate called Cassie. She is nineteen, so I'm the youngest here. Apart from us, most patients here are in there forties except for one who is fifty two. We are all female. My therapist says they don't get many men, though they do exist.

There is Sheila. She is in here for delicate cutting. She started cutting when she was forty one, so a year ago. She is from Queens and has porcelain nails. There is

Megan. She did a few that needed stitches. She doesn't do it all the time, but will do one every year or so. She has been doing it for about six years. Her three year old walked in on her once and that is why she came here. Apparently her son was in shock for a few days.

Then there is Sue-Ann who is an alcoholic, a schizophrenic, a great mom and a big cutter. She once put an electric knife inside her. Now she can't have kids again. She says it all got scrambled.

Then there is Nancy. She is the oldest and the shortest. She has ripped out two fingers on one hand and half her arm. She is constantly making jokes about Calvin. She will stick her tongue out and lick her deformed arms when he looks at her. She will pretend to blush and stutter. I think she is going to rape him one of these days.

Then there is Davina. She pours cleaning products on her legs. Well she used to now she is a cutter. God knows how someone can go from acid to a razor. She has to do it every day though. Well until she came in here. She is probably the most normal one here. No disorders apart from cutting.

There are a few others that I don't know too well, and have no wish to. They are so boring, and I never hear them speak. It's a much smaller group than at the last place, but I like it so far.

The Professionals: My psychiatrist there was a woman with a name so long that I couldn't remember it if I really tried. She was nice enough. She was very into drugs and medication. I felt like I was in an antidepressant candy store. I could take a pick a mix bag and shovel in what pills and capsules I wanted. With too much candy you get a tummy ache. With too many pills your tits lactate. When I left I had no longer heavy pads on my wrists or arms but on my breasts inside my bra instead.

19/06/01

We have videos and take outs on the weekend. We get papers to write all the time. We have groups all day too. So the weekends are the only times we can relax and do nothing. I get to have Dylan my scruffy teddy at night times.

We have a lot of art groups, and we do collages about our feelings. They are cool, and we can do anything we want. We play card games a lot, but nobody here knows how to play 'Palace'.

Calvin is kind of cool. It's easier talking to him than I thought it would be. The women who run the program are called Karen and Wendy. They are really nice. They listen to you and actually understand what you are talking about. The nurses here are cool as well. We all get assigned to one. Mine is called Lisa. She is nice and doesn't flip out when I talk about my voices. She doesn't give me the look when I tell her they could be real. She says anything is possible.

There is a monk who comes here. Brother Paul. He is funny. I have never met a monk in my life. He is in his late twenties and is a virgin. I can't believe it. Megan asked him if he had ever seen God. He said no. She told him if he were to fuck a girl he would come close to heaven.

He said that there are other ways to have pleasure. I couldn't stop laughing. We were trying to shock him. We were not successful. He has heard all the monk jokes already.

He gave us lots of gossip on catholic priests in his church, we loved it. He told us that some of the monks would sleep with their hands behind their backs. Then when they woke up they were numb. Then they could wank and imagine it was a girl's hand. That's when he was asked to leave the unit. He'll come back though.

He thought my voices were evil. He scared the shit out of me. But he was cool anyway. He watches TV and likes pop music. My idea of a monk's life was very different from how he described his. Nancy tried to seduce him. I thought that was mean. But it was hysterical too. He was like a male Whoopi Goldberg in sister act. He was a regular guy, except for the whole flip flops and robe thing. In winter he's allowed to wear sneakers.

The Regular Staff: The nurses who I saw everyday were friendly and supportive. They seemed to really know what I and the other patients were going through, although none of us knew if it was because they understood it on a personal level or not. There was one nurse to every three patients and everyday we would have a check up time where we could privately talk about how our day went with her. They would also give us assignments, which showed that every staff member who worked there was helping in our treatment.

A REASON

Then my life was in pieces, and I was bleeding. I was crying for your help. Inside I was screaming. I was trapped inside a hole. A psychiatric unit, where they left me was suffocating. My pain was so deep. I could relate to no one, except to my horror the worse of cases. Then I didn't think I could go on. Do I feel like that now? You want a positive answer, so you can tick the box entitled sane. Ask me tomorrow. I'm too scared to answer now.

20/06/01
My stomach has been acting up today. I've been sick a lot. I think it's because they have me on lots of medication. Lisa said they were going to have a look at it with a camera soon. I'm dreading it. I have not had any urges to cut today. When we do we are supposed to write them down as soon as possible. They don't mind me writing in my journal either. They say it's very

good to express myself on paper. That's a first. I have always had to hide it before.

I had a good talk with my mom today. I haven't heard from my sister for a while though. I'm starting to trust the staff in here a bit more. I no longer think that Calvin is going to hurt me, or the nurses are against me. I like all the patients too.

The Other Patients: Every patient on the unit was a self-harmer. Some had huge scars on what seemed like every part of the body, where others showed none. There were some in there for minor bodily harm and then there were those who wouldn't give a second thought to removing their eyes, genitals or setting certain body parts alight. However every patient there was treated the same no matter how minor or severe their harming was. There were only a maximum of about eleven women on the entire unit. Men were allowed there but not so many were admitted to the unit as self harm is a more female self destructive method. I got on with every patient there and was amazed at how for the first time I could relate so much to people. For the first time I didn't feel out of place.

21/06/01

Today has been weird. I've only just noticed it's been a while since the last time I wrote. Maybe because I can openly say things in group and not have to write it all secretly down. My voices haven't been around for a few days. I wonder if me getting better is scaring them off. I can sense they are weakening.

I have just come up from the recovery room downstairs. The sedatives are wearing off. They stuck two tubes in me, one up my butt and one down my throat. They put the needle thing in my hand and kept injecting more liquid every time I whined. When they stuck the tube down my throat they took pictures and I could see the inside on a large TV screen. It was disgusting. It hurt a lot. When they put it in down my throat, I thought I was going to die. I had to take my tongue piercing out. All I was worried about was if it would heal, as I took them an hour or so.

This morning I had to drink a gingery drink that I kept throwing up. Then they made me drink another one and then I had to have a shot in my but to stop me puking. It was horrid.

Departure: I stood outside on the street with my mother waiting for a taxi in the hot Chicago sun. Wendy and Karen the program directors came outside the two front doors, waved and then went around the corner for a cigarette, which I thought was funny. My mother was cursing at the fact that no taxi was in sight, would be in sight soon, or would ever be in sight at all. I looked up the towering building to try and peek into any windows. I couldn't. They were all reflecting the sun and looked like mirrors. I watched the people on the street walking past. They did not know who I was or the fact that the girl they where passing had once wanted to end her life by jumping out onto the very pavement they were walking on. The building to them could have been a block of offices for all they knew. A group of guys passed me buy, one winked at me. They did not know I was once put away for being a threat to society and myself.

22/06/01
My moods have been weird. One minute I'm happy the next I'm angry. I'm starting to remember some things from my childhood. I don't want to remember. I have been disassociating again. I haven't done that for a while.

Every one can go down to the cafeteria to eat but me. I'm not an adult yet. Some women sleep off the unit too. I can't do that either. It sucks. The night nurses are not as nice as the ones here during the day. When Cassie goes I will be the only one left here during the night. That will be so boring. Hopefully she won't go for a few weeks.

My View on the Place: Overall I believe that the
S.A.F.E program in Chicago is the best treatment
centre that I have been to or heard of, that deals with
self harm. This is because that is the primary focus of
what they deal with. The directors knew exactly what
they were dealing with and created an excellent
program that in my view is the best one there is. If I
knew someone with problems in that area I wouldn't
hesitate to recommend Chicago to them. It is a shame
that more treatment centres in England do not use
them as an example of how much help a self harmer
can get.

23/06/01
Everything has gone wrong. Yesterday was awful; I
came very close to being violent. A girl called Lori got
restrained. It wasn't pleasant. Young guys in white
uniforms, those black shoes and black belts shining.
They had their gloves on and their watches were taken
off in case they got caught on something. There was no
bed though, and no injection. My therapist helped them
carry her head. She was taken to another unit because
she was suicidal. When she was better they said they
would discharge her. She was eighteen. Adult
psychiatric would welcome her with open arms.

I got really angry. They told me they didn't restrain
anyone here. Like always I believed them. Then I got
angry, very angry. I threatened a lot of people I
shouldn't have. They were people who could lock me
up like my therapist, the nurses, and a man who had
restrained her. I yelled at Chris. I spat; I hissed I tried
so hard not to hurt him. My voices were screaming at
me, I tried to block them out. I couldn't. Then he sat
down. This time it wasn't funny like when Matt in Idaho
did it. You can always tell if someone is used to
patients like me. They don't yell back at you, or scare
you. They try and come across as non-threatening. It
made me feel safe. I get worse when I am with
someone who doesn't know how to control me. The
way a scared dog will only bite if he senses you are
nervous.

136

I didn't hurt him. I hurt myself instead. It wasn't deep. It wasn't very bad, but it was bad enough to be discharged. I'm on probation now. I can't go to groups. I have to sit here until tomorrow, until they decide what to do to with me.

The other patients are afraid of me now; just when I had built their trust. No matter how fucked up patients are they always seem scared of me. I'm harmless!

How It Affected Me: When I look back at my time spent in Chicago on the unit I believe it was a positive experience. It gave me greater insight into my disorder. Although I jeopardised my time there by breaking the contract and self harming there isn't a day that goes by that I don't regret it. To think of how much better off I would have been if I had spent my entire program on the unit is overwhelming. I still use some of their coping methods to this day and try and follow all the things the program taught me.

I AM NOT HERE

My eyes are listening to you,
But my mind is never here,
My smile a sweet deception,
Of intense and endless fear.

IT BURNS

A new experiment,
An indescribable desire,
To take a hot light bulb,
That burns like fire.
Then a horrid sensation,
Hissing and popping of skin,
Whimpering in agony,
Burning up the pain within.
A red rash of blisters,
Stinging spreading up my arm,

137

The hot glass pressed even harder,
My new way to harm.
Sleepless nights crying,
An ongoing pain,
My flesh hot and swollen,
Yet I do it again.
Yellow liquid spilling,
All the ice cubes in the world couldn't soothe,
Perhaps I'll go back to cutting,
As I only have skin to lose.

PRE-TEEN CUTTING

I sat in the school toilets,
Blood had stained the floor,
I was skipping class again,
And causing a big uproar,
Teachers were calling me,
I wanted to be alone,
It was safe inside my bubble,
I wanted to cut to the bone,
The only way to express,
My feelings deep inside,
I hated any attention,
So under long sleeves they'd hide,
In my pencil case; my life support,
Was my life long friend,
A shiny, blue plastic razor,
I'd cherish to the end,
My love for symmetrical scars,
And the designs on my arm,
I was so young then,
Didn't know it's name; self harm.

COME UNDONE

Make me bleed,
So I know I'm real,
Make me bleed,
So that I can feel. Make me bleed,
I'm so unsure,
Make me bleed,

It is the only cure.

Stitches doctor's done,
They have come undone,
This isn't fun,
I can't go on.

Make me bleed,
So I can scream,
Make me bleed,
It's what I need.
Make me bleed,
I want to cry,
Make me bleed,
So I can die.

Stitches doctor's done,
They have come undone,
This isn't fun,
I can't go on.

Make me bleed,
Use a knife,
Make me bleed,
End my life.
Make me bleed,
Stop the pain,
Make me bleed,
I need stitches again.

Stitches doctor's done,
They have come undone,
This isn't fun,
I can't go on.

Make me bleed,
Rip the black threads,
Make me bleed,
Until I'm dead.

THE SCALPEL

A glint in the silver,
Then a splash of red,
The voices screaming,
In my head.
Some scarlet tears,
Bitter and sour,
Still they scream,
My soul they will devour.
Symbols on skin,
Lines, circles a star,
Glinting silver cuts deeper,
Perhaps I've gone too far.
Falling back on my pillow,
Relaxing in pleasure full pain,
Blood drenching sheets,
Stains remain the same.
I want to disappear,
While I lie on this bed,
Hoping in the morning,
That I will wake up dead.

FRAGILE GIRL

A tear rolls from my cheek,
As it falls I catch it in my hand,
So small this salty single drop,
Yet there is so much to understand.
Within it's watery appearance,
Outlines of a young girl's portrait,
This bitter tasting puddle,
Already knows her fate.
Body young and underdeveloped,
But there is maturity in her eyes,
Her innocent childhood has been taken,
She holds secrets behind her smile.
This tiny tear is so desperate,
And sadness is all that it tastes,
Spoiled on a girl so fragile,
Its meaning has gone to waste.

As I hold her reflection in my palm,
I wonder where she calls home,
In pain all too soon I realise,
This tear is mine, this portrait my own.

LETTER FROM SELF HARM

I helped you scratch and cut,
I helped you burn,
And every scar you own,
I helped you earn,
I am whatever instrument you use,
I am the smile on your skin,
And I help you let out,
The pain bottled up within,
You can find me anywhere,
If you just look hard enough,
Your nails, blunt scissors or a rock,
Anything that's sharp or tough,
I've been with you for ages,
I help you cry red tears,
I fed off your emotions,
I'll be with you through the years,
For every second of every day,
I'll be sitting in your brain,
To push you over the edge,
Make sure you do it again,
But don't think of stopping,
You could never turn a friend away,
Besides you're too weak to last,
So with you I will stay,
On every razors edge,
You will see my reflection,
And with every blood flow,
You will feel my affection,
I control you, I own you,
You are nothing without me,
If you think you can stop,
Then try it,
But I will never set you free.

CHAPTER SEVEN

Chicago-2 Adult Psychiatric Unit.

July-August
17 Years Old

Arrival: I had just been asked to leave the self harmer's unit. I was to be put on probation and had to stay somewhere else until I was allowed back. I was led by my therapist down corridors. I had my teddy in one hand and held his hand with the other. He looked worried which made me worried. He told me I would be treated well on my new unit but I wouldn't have nominated him for an Oscar performance. He lied very badly considering his job. I entered the unit and was met by looks of interest by people who seemed truly insane. A nurse searched me and my belongings before pushing me into a two-bedroom. My bed was one of those that you see on hospital dramas. There was an old woman on the other one. She had her wrists and ankles strapped down and was yelling a man's name over and over. She had dribble down the side of her mouth and I dreaded spending the night with her.

First impression: I was scared. For the first time in my life I actually really feared for my life. What was worse was that no one knew I was there. I couldn't call out to my mum, or manipulate my doctor. My child like smile didn't fool the nurses and my defensive body language didn't frighten off the other patients on the unit. I knew now what it was like to sit in a room full of insane people. I was in a state of uncontrollable fear. I felt sick, I was shaking and I was sweating. I tried my best to look as if I blended in. I was a sheep let lose in a den of wolves and all I could do was estimate how much time I had before they would harm me.

I've been put in a nut ward again. It's horrible. They have made a mistake. I am in with the adults, but I am only seventeen. I am in a bedroom. There is an old

142

woman tied down to her bed who keeps yelling out "Jimmy!" at the top of her lungs. I am sitting behind my bed. There is screaming out side in the day room and the alarm is ringing so I guess there is a restraint.

When I got here they searched my stuff. They then strip searched me. I got told to wait in the day room. I did. Everyone here looks really scary. There is a black woman called Honey who is from Harlem. She has decided to be my bodyguard and immediately started mothering me. She is in here for trying to kill her husband. She has a court date coming up soon.

I was sitting at the table playing cards when a young guy called Johnny came up to me. He asked how old I was and my name. Then all of a sudden he started crying and said he had to tell me something. He said long distant relationships didn't work, and he had to brake up with me. I was like what the fuck are you talking about?! Honey said he was nuts. I would have to agree. He is awaiting a court date before being locked up.

It seems that every one here is waiting for a court date but me. They come here because they are too fucked up to be put in jail. All of them are going to a nut house for a long time.

There is another black guy who is in a wheel chair. He has a lazy eye and a fake hand. He brags that it isn't his good hand so he can still wank. Most of the patients here are men. They all came up to me like I was the only girl they have seen in a long time.

One big guy who kept dribbling grabbed me and then an anorexic grabbed me too. Then they started to get into my clothes. I was shouting for the nurse, who never came. Honey attacked them, and I ran to my room. She said they just needed to get laid.

I wish I could call someone. I don't know how long I will be here. I am not allowed to use the phone. I can't remember any numbers. If I did I would call Mc Phillips and offer him thousands to come get me, but I can't. I am stuck in a nut unit again just because I cut.

I am too scared to leave my room. This fucking woman won't shut up. The guys keep trying to get into my room. This big Tec stops them. I don't want to spend the night here. I want to kill myself. Maybe I can find something sharp and slit my wrists.

The Professionals: I didn't ever see a psychiatrist on that unit, nor did I see a therapist, social worker or mental health technician.

The Regular Staff: There were two nurses on the entire unit, one male one female. Both of them seemed to hate their jobs. Both seemed to hate the patients because of who they were. Although I pointed out several times that I was not like them, they hated me anyway as well. They would both make fun of the elderly patients and tease the ones that they new could not hurt them. The nurses would both make sexual comments about some and openly laugh at the others.

The Other Patients: The patients on that unit were all in there as a temporary solution while they waited for sentencing. Some would go to prison but most would be placed into a psychiatric hospital after their court trials and cases were over with. There was a mixture of both sexes but the majority were male. Their ages ranged from twenty nine to eighty one. I was the only one who was not an adult. A mistake made by lost paper work. Most of the patients were in there for rape or murder. Some had sexually assaulted minors where others had done it to their own children. They seemed to live in their own little world most of the time. Occasionally when realising where they were they would try committing suicide and quite badly in my opinion. They would do it in front of everyone. There was no imagination in it at all. It was not an art for them but a simple way of demanding attention from the staff. On the unit there were probably about twenty five

144

patients. Some were very aggressive towards everyone others were physically abusing patients. There was not one restraint while I was there. The staff seemed to let the patients sort out there differences on their own, like dogs in a park. In general they were the sort of people that if you saw them on the streets you would walk quickly to the other side and hope they wouldn't follow you home. They were the type you saw in movies about crazy patients and the kind of people who you saw on the news and thanked god that they had been put away.

Departure: I had been fetched back by Calvin my therapist. He had rushed through the doors like a superhero and in about a minute he had picked my stuff and me up and run out of the unit with me. The relief was overwhelming. A bit like when you need the bathroom and have to wait for hours. First there is such desperation and panic and then there is pure bliss. That is how I felt.

A SECRET PLACE

There is a place where the mad go. It's a secret place between the living and the dead. The crazy, disturbed, psychotic, and the sad linger there. It's a place where no normal living person can cross over to, no matter how hard he or she try. People read, study and try to understand the state of those that live in that world. They can come close. Sometimes too close. Yet they will never fully understand.

At times I find myself in that lost world. I am given two choices. I either choose to lead a life in between the normal world and that place. Constantly drifting, or to die. Those that live in a normal world chose life. In this dark place, death is the favoured optio but it becomes an obsession.

Everything you see screams out what it could be used for: Knife-death, rope-death, pills-death, river-death, bridge-death, gun-death, HIV-death. This is until it overwhelms you to the point where you wonder if gauging out your eyes would be better.

My View on the Place: Had I not seen it I would have never believed it. If I had heard about it from a friend I would immediately presume that they had been exaggerating to make their story more exciting. I would have expected it on a documentary that wanted to shut it down but not on a floor of a well respected hospital in Chicago. I think it is sad that this is all these people get while waiting for their verdict. Even though some of the patients a part of me wanted to see rot in hell when I heard what they had done, there were others who I truly felt sorry for. The hatred the staff had for them was so inhuman and cold, even though by instinct they felt that way. The patients on that unit would eventually have been punished by laws, but I didn't feel it necessary for the staff to take on that role before their trial was over. It was one of the most unprofessional units I have ever seen.

How It Affected Me: I had to use every life skill and all my judgement of personalities if I wanted to last an hour among them. It was one of the shortest but most frightening experiences of my life. Even though I hated being on that unit and find it hard to think about I have to admit to myself that a lot of positive things came out of it all. To start with it was the first time that I realised that I was not mad. I might be crazy at times but I was curable. I could be helped I was not insane. It made me have more respect for the authority figures I hated, as it was down to them that these people had been put away and stopped from harming innocent victims. It gave me more respect for myself and a sense of pride that I although scared could handle a situation where most people would curl up in a ball and wet themselves. I feel grateful that I could have had an experience that most people never will. Most importantly it gave me a wake up call. It helped me to finally understand that if I didn't work hard at my recovery and therapy I might have one day ended up like the patients in that unit. It gave me hope for myself and my life.

BELOVED KNIFE

Beloved knife,
Cut out my fear,
Stay beside me,
As I lie dying here.
Help me be strong to end my life,
Cut out my fear my beloved knife.
Let your blade make me bleed,
You know what I need.
Let me die,
Let this be the end,
My beloved knife,
My only friend.
Let loose a deep red tear,
Then with passion cut out my fear.
I am young,
But there is no point to my life,
I beg you to kill me,
My beloved knife.
Your sharp silver edge,
So perfect so clear,
Cut out my fear.
With a twist end my life,
Help me to die,
My beloved knife.

ALL ALONE

In here from the world we hide,
Locked rooms to keep us inside,
The doctors here never show,
Other staff members don't want to know.

They control us with intense fear,
Screaming and crying we all hear,
Some minds o.k., some are gone,
The fact that I'm a patient is wrong.

My only escape can't heal,
It is a flame or a piece of steel,
I cut skin and fat not to the bone,
We are all held here alone.

NO MEMORY

This always happens,
Something has triggered it off,
I feel I'm in a nightmare,
I can't get out I'm lost,
How long have I done this?
As far as I can remember,
Someone is screaming at me,
Will it be like this forever?
They are claiming I did some things,
Violent, disturbed and cruel,
I guess I did them,
I'll have to leave this school,
I hurt someone close to me,
Tried to set her on fire,
When I say I can't remember,
They just call me a fucked up liar.

CHAPTER EIGHT

Chicago 3: Adolescent Psychiatric Unit

July-August
17 years old

Arrival: I felt like I was the odd one out again. Everyone on the unit didn't look a day over fourteen, even though they tried desperately too. It looked like a normal unit to me. On the way in I saw the restraint room, and a seclusion room. The nursing station was positioned so that every room could be seen from the desk. There were the mirrors in the corner so you could see around every bend. I was more relaxed. Everyone seemed quiet and pleasant.

First Impression: the nurses were young women. They had colourful printed nursing tops on and girly braids in their hair. Most of them were wearing lip gloss and they spoke softly. The patients didn't pose a threat to me. I thought it was funny that I was in there with them after what I had just come from. I had plans within five minutes of arriving of who I could manipulate and how I could hide the things they would not allow me to have. Everyone seemed to not be experienced with Borderlines. I was in heaven; I knew I could wrap them all around my finger. I settled in quickly.

I have been moved at last. I am so happy. A few hours ago I was in the adult nut unit. Then Calvin came running through the doors and told me to grab my stuff. He said it was all a mistake. I almost cried I was so happy. I didn't say goodbye to anyone, I just ran and didn't stop running. I thought I would go back to the old ward but I didn't. He took me through loads of corridors and then took me here. Then he left. I didn't know where I was for ages. Then I realised. It was adolescent psychiatric. I wasn't happy but it was better than the adult unit.

Everyone here is like me. They have voices, they get violent, they cut, and they try to kill themselves. They did a check on me and I had to hide my tongue piercing. If they would have seen it they would have taken it, and it would have closed up. It is also good to keep because if I need to cut then I can use it.

The staff here are really patronising. They obviously hate their jobs and don't bother hiding it. Like the adult unit most are going to be here for a short while before being passed onto a permanent place.

It sucks here. We get to sleep in but we have a group every day from 9:00am to 1:00pm. That's four hours! It's hell. No one is allowed to speak but the staff. They lecture us on why we need to be in here and how we are hurting our families. They don't know shit.

The rest of the day we do nothing at all. We sit, we sleep, and we eat. There are 2 to 1. Which means two nurse's to every patient. We can't discuss why we are here, so nobody knows anything. Everyone gets his or her own room and a nurse sits outside.

There are some patients who just sit like zombies. They stare out the window and twitch. They look really freakish. There are some very young patients, like four or five who watch cartoons all day. I don't understand what's wrong with them.

There is a little boy who goes around punching some people, including me. If you tell him not to he will bend his head back and howl for ages. The nurses do nothing but give him a shot. Then he is quiet for a while. I have never heard him speak.

The Professionals: I saw my old psychiatrist who gave me more medication to help me recover from the trauma of being on the last unit. She upped my dose of sleeping pills and gave me an emergency prescription for when I needed it. She would babble on about why I was on my medications and I would contemplate whether to hide the meds high up under my lip or at the base of my throat behind my tonsils.

I had a dream last night of Lucy a friend of mine from one of the schools I had been to. I wondered what she was up to now. I wondered if she knew where I was, I had suddenly disappeared and I couldn't remember who I had told. She must know I am losing my memory. I had known her since I was eight years old. Her mother was my doctor and I often stayed at her house while my mother was in London. She came to Sweden with me once. It was in the summer. We were about fifteen years old. We had gone to an outdoor gig. We had danced for hours and gotten really drunk on champagne and red wine. That night I had been introduced to my dad's girlfriend and I had been so upset. I drank to forget. We had been right in front of the stage and my eardrums felt like they had exploded. We had kicked off our shoes. The ground was muddy and slippery. We were hot and sweaty. My sister Kat was there too. She was twelve, I think. We loved it. We danced weirdly as if no one was watching and I couldn't stop laughing. Kat was laughing too. Her forehead was frowned and she had tears running down her cheeks. She held her tummy in pain. We all hugged each other and pulled funny faces to the rest of the crowd. We checked out the guys that were there and took in the deep smell of the woods and fern bushes that were around us. I was so happy to have Lucy on holiday with me, as I valued her friendship the most. I trusted her more than any other classmate because she had always been there for me and I knew somehow she always would.

In a few hours the gig was over and yet we were still there dancing. Everyone had gone home but we wanted to claim the night and hold on to the moment. The singer and musicians had left and some lads were starting to dismantle the stage and all the lighting equipment. It needed to be taken down by sunrise. Lucy and I grabbed a pole each that had supported part of the stage. We started dancing for the guys. I had run out of cigarettes and needed some more. I begged the guys for some and followed one man to his car pleading him for a fag. He rolled me one and I remember choking on the strength of the nicotine. I resumed my dancing and Kat applauded Lucy and I as we did our ridiculous moves that we thought were so sexy and cool. My hands hurt and my hair was a mess. I felt dizzy and the stars in the sky seemed to blend into one big painting. I felt so alive and so loved. I was so angry that my dad had been such a bastard and stayed with his girlfriend all night. I was furious at him and felt sorry for me and my sister. So I kept twirling round my pole and I sung an Aerosmith song over and over again that had stuck in my head all day. "Pink," I sang, "It was love at first sight, pink when I turn out the light, pink gets me high as a kite, and I think everything is going to be alright no matter what we do tonight."

The Regular Staff: I didn't get to know the regular staff that well apart from one nurse who I manipulated very well. Now I should have got an Oscar. I managed to hide my tongue stud throughout my entire stay. Even when showing my mouth open when getting my medication. I would put the bottom ball of my steel bar in front of my bottom teeth behind my lip, and that would create a groove in my tongue that in the right light hid the top ball. My tongue would appear flat when it was not. Inside this dip was also a good place to hide a small pill. The nurses were obviously not that well trained or they would have spotted this immediately. The nurses didn't seem to like their jobs on this unit either though and seemed to treat me and the other patients like children. Even though we were, but they would talk to us as if we were five years old rather than young adults.

Wendy came to see me today. She explained I am here because I had scared a lot of patients on the ward. She told me that once I have written several papers and proven I am not violent, I could come back. I never thought I had scared anyone. I now feel guilty and want to cut. If I do I can't go back to the ward at all. I have to try very hard.

I hope I can go back soon. There is nothing to do here. There is a dodgy man who is my 24 hour. He won't stop staring at me. When I ask him to stop, he say's it's his job.

The Other Patients: most of the patients on the unit used self harm as a way of coping, but now that I look back at my time spent there I feel they did it more to get attention rather than as a coping method. They were a lot like the teenagers that I saw in boot camp. I wouldn't go as far as to say that they were mentally ill but they did however have some issues that I could relate to. I thought it was humorous to watch patients claim that they were grown up, but then go and watch the Lion King on the television.

My voices have been bad all day. I missed group because I was disassociating. They said they don't like to interrupt when that happens in case I get angry. I have never heard that before. They act as if I was in a board meeting.

I had to sit through a boring video today. Some dumb cartoon, I had seen several times. My wrist hurts. I have been writing all afternoon on my assignments. I hope I can leave here soon.

THE BEDROOMS

There were ten bedrooms. Each one had three beds inside that were basic wooden frames nailed down to the floor, and the plastic covered mattresses which made squelching noises every time someone moved on them. The bathrooms had the locks cut out and the shower curtains removed, "just in case," the staff would say when we complained.

I never worried about showering naked hoping no one would come in like most patients did. I had to have a 24 hour on me. Meaning whatever I did, where ever I went I had to have a nurse a meter away at all times, except for when in the time out room.

Departure: I was happy to be going back to my old unit and to join my old therapy groups. I was also nervous about what the other patients thought of me after I was off probation. I felt that I had jeopardised their recovery, which in fact I had done.

There is a guy called Bobby in here. I don't know what he is in for. He was meant to leave today. They came to collect him. He thought he was going home. The staff told him he was going to another place for a long time. He attacked a nurse. I have never seen a kid so young react like that. He scratched at her eyes and she was screaming. He bit her very hard. She was swearing at him. He got put in restraint. Then a few other kids joined in. They were all so small!

One little boy who has been banging his head since he arrived, started thumping himself really hard. Soon everyone but me was doing something. Then the alarm was called and the restraint men came running. I ran to my room and hid.

In the end six of the patients got restrained and four got put in time out rooms to calm down. Only myself, and a guy called Toby were not hurt. Nurses and patients were seen too for their scratches. They put me in time out. I don't know why. They said it was for my safety. I was only in there for an hour.

Most patients got taken to other wards because this one didn't have enough rooms. It was so funny to see everyone suddenly gang up on the staff. I guess they were bored. There isn't much to do around here but piss them off. They don't handle it well.

My View on the Place: It was not a place where I would have made goals or made any good progress into handling my behaviour. The staff were too inexperienced and treated it more like a summer job than a serious career. Many times they didn't know how to handle a situation or deal with a rebellious patient.

How It Affected Me: It didn't affect me a great deal nor did it teach me anything I did not already know. I realised that I was good at manipulating staff members and that I could often get my own way, but none of those things were new to my knowledge. In my opinion it was a waste of time and money but it was the only option for me to stay while I was not allowed back onto the unit I was meant to be in.

A SAFE PLACE

Most of us hated the hospital, but we knew we needed it too. We were not part of the real world any more, the one that had made us crazy. We had been put away into a place where society could forget about us, and where normal people didn't have to worry that we lived in their towns and cities. They felt safe knowing we were locked up.

What most people on the outside didn't realise was that it was a relief to be kept away from them. We now no longer had to worry about the demands and expectations of the world. Inside the only thing expected of us was that we were ill. As long as we remained sad, psychotic, morbid, and disturbed we could stay as long as we wanted.

We did not have to worry about school, our families or getting jobs. We were free and had nothing to lose. Everything we had had been taken from us. Our privacy, our dignity, and respect were all gone. Yet at

155

the same time we had every thing we ever needed.
The hospital provided food that was edible enough, and
scrubs as clothes. They provided us a home where we
were understood. When we arrived they stripped us
clean of everything and then they sheltered us.

INSANE NEEDS

Soft and gentle kisses,
Then a punch to my head,
I wondered if you would leave me there,
Wishing I were dead.
A followed sweet apology,
All I could ask was why,
Then pining down flesh on flesh,
Warning me not to cry.
Carefully planning your blows,
Knowing not to bruise the face,
Craving ropes and leather,
Ripping silk and lace.
Excuses well rehearsed,
Prepared for when it happens again,
Thoughts racing through my mind,
In case wounds I must explain.
You knew I was fragile,
That I thought I'd never be free,
And if I ever spilled your secret,
No one would believe me.
A sudden switch of mood,
You're craving for a blood spilling game,
Your fucked up sexual urges,
Those were illegal and insane.

OUR SECRET GAME

It first began with touches,
Then into your world I fell,
You called it our secret game,
I swore I'd never tell.
I knew where to touch,
You taught me phrases to say,

I learnt how to make a man smile,
From our game we would play.
Then things started changing,
Our game got very rough,
You told me to stay silent,
To take it and be tough.
The first time there was ripping,
It burnt like fire inside,
Told me to be quiet,
You got mad because I cried.
I thought it was a one off,
But you wanted it again and again,
It was from you I realised,
That love was linked with pain.
Our game went on for years,
And then a sudden stop,
There was no interest once I'd hit puberty,
I tried to forget but could not.
You taught me important things,
How to please a man in every way,
I was left permanently scarred,
From the games we would play.

INFINITE AGONY

With you I got pulled down,
From the ledge of sanity I fell,
I wasn't happy, but surviving,
Now I'm condemned to your world of hell,
You grabbed the advantage of my youth,
I was searching, I was blind,
With your madness, you fed,
The devils that danced in my mind,
You spun a web of darkness,
Around my confused existence,
After punishing, came apology,
An evil that lacked all sense,
Thoughts of love and hate entangled,
Angelic eyes with a morbid grin,
If only you knew my infinite agony,
Each time you forced yourself deep within.

CHAPTER NINE

Kent - Treatment Centre

August-November
17-18 years old

Arrival: It was a long drive from our home. My mother was driving me. I had been chain smoking for almost three hours so the old Volvo stunk of stale nicotine. My throat was sore, as usual we had spent the time singing to our favourite songs as loud as our voices would allow. My mother tried to rap like Eminem and looked so sweet trying to be cool. She had informed me that I would not be able to have any medication, caffeine or sugar while I was there. Having taken several pills in the morning I then resulted in scoffing down doughnuts, chocolate and crisps and a two-litre coke bottle. I managed to get the majority of my soon to be confiscated sweets on the car interior. My legs were sticky with dried cola and I had jam down my t-shirt. My mother who is an official chocoholic claimed she would have "just one" of everything. But soon just one turned into a full blown binge session that left us exhausted and our trousers unbuttoned.

16/08/01. 11:56pm
I'm at the new program and I hate it. I am worried because they don't let me have any meds here. They are really against any prescription drugs. I think the staff here are so fucked up.

My voices are back and they are freaking me out. I cut myself again and I am not going to tell the staff. I arrived late so I didn't have to do any groups at all which was a relief.

It took three hours to drive here and the whole way I was feeling sick I was so nervous. It seemed to take forever. It looks like a large private house, but it looks too nice. There are no barred windows. They don't

158

have any restraints, but thinking of some patients here they should.

I have to share a bedroom with three other patients. I hate sharing. Everyone here seems to be addicts. They have one girl called Abby who is a cutter but that's it.

First Impression: When we finally arrived it looked like a large manor house. I felt funny about it at the start. But maybe that was the meds I'd swallowed desperately earlier. I didn't like it and my gut instinct was to run. To please my mother I didn't. Well not at first. There were however no windows with bars on them and they didn't have any seclusion rooms. The grounds were pretty and it seemed as if a patient could just walk off into the fields if they chose too.

17/08/01 10:08pm.
Today was horrible. I have been throwing up and so I had to miss several groups. A nurse said she had cut down my meds too fast. I have also been feeling really dizzy and I keep getting panic attacks for no reason.

A counsellor here called Lillian let me talk to my mom, which wasn't much help, all she did was scream at me for ages. I agreed that I would go back to Chicago if she got me out of here. She said she would come and pick me up tomorrow.

There is a girl here called Connie. She has a limp on her left leg. Dr. R the guy who runs this place told the group that she tried to kill herself. She jumped out a seven story floor window and landed onto concrete. She was fine except for her leg. That's pretty cool. She is really weird though.

18/08/01 9:44pm.
Today was so fucked up. My mum never came because Dr. R had called her and told her not to. He is such a cult leader. They just brainwash everyone here. I think he is so fucked up in the head.

I ran away and tried to call some friends to come get me but kept running out of money. I tried to hitch hike but there were no cars. This place is in the middle of nowhere. When I was back at the program I got yelled at. I cut myself in the shower really badly and my voices are bugging the hell out of me. I wish I had some medication for them!

24/08/01 11:52pm.
I just did my step one for cutting. Its so stupid cutting is not an addiction it is a coping method. The doctor here isn't even a psychiatrist. He thinks anything and everything is an addiction, he is so clueless. He has an answer for everything I hate people like that.

Today is Friday and on Sunday we can have visitors. Then I can get some more clothes and some more fags. I don't want to leave anymore but I still don't like it here. I am just going to deal with it instead.

On Thursday I had to do this walk with the rest of the group. I was walking behind with Malcolm. My shoes gave me really bad blisters and I got very pissed off. Apparently when patients leave here they then go down to London to stay at a half way house, but I will probably be here for ages before that.

The girl with the limp has gone. Her parents came and took her. I think that they put her into psychiatric.

The Professionals: The doctor who ran the place seemed nice at first. He acted as if he genuinely wanted to help me. He persisted in trying to convince me that I was an addict not a Borderline. He thought that self harming like everything else was an addiction and not a behaviour. He was very active in the patient's recovery and we saw him for a three hour therapy group everyday. He was on the grounds most of the day so we could talk to him whenever we wanted to. I did however question his views from the start. He was good in his intentions but I feel that he was far more interested in getting his money and being interviewed on television than what the patients were feeling.

02/09/01, 11:55pm
My mum came today and went to the family group and to one of Dr. R's lectures. I guess that some are all right but he goes on so much that I lose concentration after about five minutes.

I sat in the car for hours listening to music and ran the battery out. Mike had to come and help us restart it. Fiona is leaving tomorrow. I'm going to miss her. She always makes everyone smile.

Everyone is very tense or sad today. Caroline broke up with Alex and cut herself for the first time. That pissed me off as she only did it for attention.

I am still cutting but I never tell anyone when I do it. And I choose to do it in places where they can't see. I don't understand why they think it is a problem. I can stop whenever I want to; I just don't want to stop. People tell me that I can't control it. They don't understand. It is the only thing that I can control. And I won't do it for the rest of my life. It is just the only way I can cope with things.

I called Karl today. He has relapsed again. He told me that Steve from London 2 hospital had died of an overdose.

06/09/01, 11:09pm
Today was all right. It was fairly boring. I have a new roommate and she is really sweet. I cut myself badly today. It was on my arm in the shower. I think it needs stitches but I can't tell anyone. I cracked open a razor and used the blade. I just wanted to shut my voices up. I am so stupid. I shouldn't have done it on my arm. Then again its winter soon so it will be getting cold. That means I can cover it up. I don't want anyone to find out.

The Regular Staff: The therapists there all believed in the doctor and his methods of dealing with addiction. They were all addicts themselves so could relate to all the patients. They were tough but they cared and did the best that they knew how to try and help the patients understand why they were there and why they had to give up their drug of choice. There were a few good staff members. They made us laugh and have a more enjoyable time. They were not as strict when not under the doctor's watchful eye and made the whole ordeal of being in rehab a bit more bearable.

16/09/01, 10:42pm

I'm in a room with Lizzy and Anne. Anne is going to leave tomorrow. Dr. R has told her if she does then she can't come back. She is very fucked up. She won't eat anything and spits out all her food. She used to be forced to give an old guy head. Now she thinks whenever she puts food in her mouth it's his cum. I think she might kill herself and there is nothing we can do. I hate the way it is here. She has been here for months and the staff have done nothing to help her at all. They don't seem to care. All the patients hate it.

18/09/01, 11:20pm

Its just under four weeks till my birthday, when I can leave for three days. I can't wait. I am going to get my lip pierced and have all my hair braided. I will be able to cut as much as I want. I am planning to use a razor, kitchen knife or scalpel.

Anne has decided to stay. The staff said she would be sectioned otherwise. Lizzy, Victoria and I had a group with her today. I couldn't handle it and walked out.

Mathew had a group today and went on and on about having a gift. He thinks he is telepathic. He is so nutty. I don't understand why the staff here have people like him in this program. It is obvious that he needs help and medication.

21/09/01, 10:37pm
My hallucinations were horrible today. About an hour
ago I went for a fag outside and I saw the white people
hanging from a tree. They were really creeping me out.
But I didn't cut. I was just screaming at the top of my
lungs for ages. I have decided that they have to be
real. I don't care what people think. If others saw them
they would think that too.

12/10/01, 11:05pm
Yesterday was really shit. A new girl called Simone
came. She is so screwed up. She thinks that the devil
possesses her. She has voices too so I had to show
her around. She wouldn't stay still but had to keep
walking around. She would suddenly start crying for no
reason and tell her voices to stop bothering her. She
said she was a protector of a little child that no one else
saw.

She started freaking me out and said that I was
possessed too. Then she got very abusive towards
everyone. She said that I was evil because I cut myself.
I was so close to beating the fuck out of her.

A therapist called a group and we all sat in a room and
had to talk about voices for ages. He is such a dick. He
was way over his head and tried to tell us that she was
an addict. Exactly what she was addicted to he never
said.

It was so obvious to everyone that she had a mental
disorder. The whole group got angry that she was to
stay in this program.

14/10/01, 12:00am
Caroline keeps going on about her cutting. She thinks
that she is in agony, but they are only paper thin. I can't
wait to get out of here. When I go to London I am going
to run away, I can't handle this place anymore.

It is starting to get a bit cooler. I had to wear a jumper in group. I played tennis today with Piers and Peter. Piers beat me though so I was annoyed at him. Later on he played the guitar for me though so I forgave him.

I saw my aunt not long ago. She has been separated from my uncle for a while now but I think that she still misses him. Every Swedish woman I know is so weak.

No one in my family stays married to the same woman. They all have to break up their families due to their dicks. All the ex wives just cry and moan. They should get them arrested, take them to court, expose them for what they are or beat them up. I can't understand women who put up with that shit. I refuse to be like that. When I have a child I will never expose them to that. I will not let certain family members go near my baby. What kind of role models are these men to children? Do they not realise what all their friends secretly think about them behind their backs? I have listened in on dinner parties and lunches; I have heard what guests in our own house have said about my dad and my uncle. Men like these are sociably accepted due to their wealth or popularity. They are no different from the addicts that are on the streets or in jail. Do they not realise that?

16/10/01, 10:20pm
It was my birthday today. I went down to London last night. My mum came into my very small bedroom singing and had some presents. There was hardly any space for her. I have a single bed and a chest of drawers in my room. That's all that will fit. I am in our flat now. It is very small and I'm not used to living in such a tiny space. Thank god my sister is not here or she would have had to sleep in my mum's bed. She is still at boarding school in the country. I liked my presents. I am bored. There is not much to do. We had to sell our larger house. I loved it. We always move from house to house and it is so unsettling.

In an hour I am going up the high street to have my hair braided. It will take six hours apparently. I am going to bring a book. It is so nice to be out of treatment. I have been in there for months and don't want to go back. I am also going to pierce my lip.

The Other Patients: Every patient there was an addict. It ranged from heroin to alcohol, to sex and love addiction or compulsive helping. One man was there for being a computer addict, another for being addicted to coffee or anything else that contained caffeine. They were all rebellious at the start but soon absolutely loved the place. There was only one other self harmer while I was there and she was sure that her cutting was an addiction. Since I left that treatment centre five people in my group are dead. Most of them overdosed as soon as they left. There are about another ten who in my opinion will die any day. Not many patients who left remained clean after leaving. Although every rehab has its death ratings I find that the one at Kent was high.

17/10/01, 11:00pm
I hate it here. I am back at the treatment centre and I have a new room mate. I have moved rooms as well so I can't get used to my bed being in a different position. Tomorrow I have to show someone around who might put their brother in here. I can't wait. I haven't shown someone round yet. Everyone else has. I don't know why they have not chosen me to do it before.

At least I am not with Caroline anymore. I really like her but her constant moaning about her true love leaving is driving me crazy. I went up to see Piers an hour ago. He has a roommate who is cool. He keeps doing really rude jokes that are so funny. It felt good to laugh.

18/10/01, 11:18pm
I had to show this woman around. She was heavily pregnant and had just flown in from Australia. She seemed fun though and her husband kept jumping on the beds to make sure that they were okay to lie on. I told her why she should put her brother in here. I lied

through my teeth about how great it was in the groups. I did however think that her brother would get better in here. Some patients should be somewhere else but I think that this place sounded right for him.

I have been playing the guitar with Caroline. Piers joined in. He is so amazing on it. He plays so well. He doesn't usually want to play for us so it was a real treat.

24/10/01, 10:06pm
A new guy is here. He is called Bob. I guess his sister liked it here because a few days ago she came to look around. He is here for over eating and compulsive helping, I think. He seems really nice. Caroline has been flirting with him but I don't think he has picked up on the signals yet. He doesn't seem to talk much. I think it is the shock of being here. I tried to talk to him but I think that he needs to be on his own for now. He has a limp. I think he has some sort of illness of the muscles but I am not sure yet.

A lot of people from the group left today. They all went down to London to be in the half way house. Harry is really upset. Two of his good mates are now gone. He seems depressed. He didn't want to talk to anyone. I chatted to him for an hour and I think I cheered him up. I gave him a massage that I then got told off for by one of the therapists. They get so paranoid. He is in here for drugs not sex addiction. I think so anyway. Maybe I shouldn't have done it. But it's not as if it is a crime.

26/10/01, 09:18pm
I can't believe what happened this afternoon. I was in the computer room and looking down onto the courtyard and I saw some new patient walk into the nursing station. They looked familiar but I couldn't think of who it was. Then I recognised her bag. It was Esther. I yelled Es at the top of my lungs but she couldn't figure out where it was coming from. I ran down all the steps until I got to the nurses office. I hugged her so hard. Now finally I can maybe enjoy this place. I hadn't seen her for months. When I left one

treatment centre in London we were in together I had lost her number and address. From the look of her she was still on smack. She was thinner than I remembered and she told me that she had finally started injecting. I paraded round with her and introduced her to everyone. The nurse said that after she had been detoxed we could share a room.

I am so excited. We have so much catching up to do. I haven't seen her for so long and it will be nice to get into trouble with someone again. Caroline and I sat in the garden with Piers after dinner. We found him as he was trying to hide away. He seemed to be annoyed that we joined him. He kept hinting that we should go. I felt bad but Caroline insisted that we stay. She wanted him so badly. Apparently he hadn't had sex for a while and this just excited her more. I thought it was so weird though as she was a virgin.

01/11/01, 05:07am

I have been so much happier now that Es is here. We have been talking about the treatments we were in before this one. She hates it here too. She likes Harry but he is HIV positive. I had to drive down to London today with a therapist to collect someone. Her name was Alice. I don't know what her problem was though. She didn't seem to be a junkie. She wasn't shaking from alcohol. In the car on the way back she seemed really scared. It was obviously her first time. She was what I call a rehab virgin. She was breathing heavily and was crying in the car. When she arrived she didn't want to meet anyone. When I told people that she was 14 years old she got very angry and told me that she was 17. I wouldn't have guessed, as she was small and childlike. I said sorry but she just went to her room.

I think that she really misses her parents and her sister. She has been showing me her piercings. She has a huge thin spike in her lip. We talked for ages and she seems so intelligent and funny. I have been sitting up with Es talking and now I am really tired. I have to be up for breakfast in two hours. Alice is in a room with me and Es. And we seem to get on perfectly.

IT TAKES TWO TO TANGO WITH DEATH

Come let us run away. I will think of an escape route and you pack a bag. Let us fly to the real world. We shall leave this hospital and start our life anew. Take me to the streets that understand me. There we will live without the watchful eyes of the doctors. We will laugh at passers by and dare each other to play pranks on them. Then we can take turns sleeping so that no one takes our stuff. If anybody tries to hurt us we will fight back with all our fury. Get out your needles, I have got a spoon. Give me that vitamin C, you stole from boots. There use that ld cigarette filter. I have the dealer's number. I've got my razor at the ready. I found it last night on the way here. It will do for now. In just moments we will share our bliss. You with your eyes so pinned and me with my blood flowing. Cook up the heroin while I prepare the sacrifice. With your drugs and my self harm we soon will be floating.

Goodbye mum and dad. This is what I have chosen to do. I am in control of my skin and flesh. It is my property and I have the final say. Quick the cops are coming, run into that back alley. There we can spend the night. We can sleep without being bothered but with the sunrising you are shaking and angry. The smack is all gone and we have no money at all. You better start begging if you want your fix because the dealers won't dish out any more freebies. There go and talk to that man. He wants to give us money. Are you scared? I will come with you. How much will he give us and for what? Wait my arm. Oh my God it is bad. It's swollen to twice the normal size. It has gone dead. I can't feel it! I can't feel my own arm! It was that rusty razor blade I used last night. I knew it was old and dirty. I found it by the roadside. You need your fix, you are getting very ill but I need to get an injection. We need to go back to the doctors and the therapists. We need to go back to that hell. Fly back with me to the ward. With broken wings

168

we will have to face the other patients. This way of life is not working, we need their help.

COMPETITION

You call that a cut? I did it worse than that before I even hit puberty. I dare you to go deeper than I just did. My turn, I will do it with this nail I managed to dig out from a chair in the family therapy room. Come on! That is nothing it looks like a paper cut. Do more, and cut down harder. I double dare you. Now it is bleeding that's better. Look at mine. That is a proper cut. That's going to really scar. Okay I win. Is that fat? I think it is muscle, shit it hurts! Quick get me that t-shirt it is bleeding far too much. Put a sanitary towel on yours and pull your bra up a bit further that will hold it in place. The doctor can't find out we did this. Practise smiling. Laugh as though you're happy and dry your eyes. It's getting dark out. It is time for the last group of the day. Let's skip it. Slide out the window. Keep your head down and run. Faster towards the cornfield they won't find us there.

We can lie and watch the stars from here. For a short while we can pretend that we are not in a treatment centre. Your stomach is rumbling. Did you not eat again today? They will section you soon. I will lie back and get the dirt in my hair. Ants crawl up my hands. You sit on an old tree stump and suck in the much needed nicotine. You cry out as a nettle burns your ankle where your trousers do not cover. We freeze in silence wondering if the nurse heard us. We are too scared to even breathe. My cut on my arm has stopped bleeding now. Your white bra is soaked in blood. Infinity passes. We are too caught up in the imaginary world. Out here we can breathe and forget who we actually are. We are inpatients for life. But we don't want to think about that now. I haven't seen the stars for so long. They seem further away than usual.

The therapist is calling our names. Run back to the room. We will sit and smile about our short time outside. We will lie and say we have been here all along working on our recovery. Hold a book in front of your chest. Your top is starting to stain. It is soon time to go to our bedrooms. Then they will never know. They will talk about us as usual tomorrow to our parents and say what great progress we are making. They will not see the secrets held on our skin.

Departure: I was tired. I had had therapy up to my eyeballs. I was a walking example of the treatment centre. I was now apparently a well-behaved addict. I had wanted to leave for what seemed like years. I was ready to move on to their secondary treatment in London. I was physically and mentally exhausted and I couldn't wait to get to the new place I would call home, just so I could get some sleep.

05/11/01, 02:08am
I am going to London very soon. I am worried about what the patients there are going to be like. Soon I will be in the real world. I will be able to walk outside when I want. I am sure that I can resist the temptations. They will be everywhere. Bob had a group today and he did really well in it. He told us of his life in Australia and his problems with food. He really was open and honest. I was so proud of him. He has gone through so much and is working so hard on his recovery. He doesn't piss and moan like the rest of us do. He stands up and faces the fact that before he was here his life needed help. He has finally realised that he needs to change and that is the first step to recovery.

We went to an A.A. meeting today. It was good. There was one woman there who was heavily pregnant. She kept going outside for fag breaks. I was outside with her and she kept moaning. I was so scared that she would go into labour. She didn't but it really worried me. I kept focusing on her instead of the meeting.

When I came back, Bob and I went to sit by E.T. We could here Pete singing the song Oklahoma, from the musical, at the top of his voice. We just laughed. It would be the last time I sat next to that E.T statue. I think a past patient had made it. It looked so funny standing there at the edge of the neat garden. I thought I was hallucinating the first time I saw it. We sat there Bob and me and we giggled about things we did in our past that we thought were normal but were obviously not. Time seemed to stop for a while. It stood still for a few moments so that we could for once laugh at life. If you lay back and closed your eyes and let all the sounds around you drain away, then just for a couple of minutes you wouldn't know you were in a rehab. You would be a regular kid, one who laughs and has no worries. One who had their life ahead of them and was still naive at to what the real world was like. You would just feel like a normal person, who was exchanging jokes with a good friend.

06/11/01, 01:20am
Sam had come back for a group. He had been playfully winding up Lillian. He had chased Caroline and me around the garden. He sat for ages and stroked the cats. He loved them, but I was a dog person. He had a hat on, like a beanie and kept trying to get the cat to wear it. I was grumpy. I had attempted to stop smoking without much success. Piers has been jumping in puddles all today. He showed me a picture of his niece, which I got all broody over, she was so cute. We argued over who was the better skier, him or me.

I was feeling a bit down so he cheered me up by coming up with a long, lengthy and very detailed story of some blue African elephants who went on holiday to meet their cousins in India, who by the way were pink. Then they, the blue elephants, became warriors and were fighting these weird people called the Moollies who all had terribly weird names like king Theodore Gorthengarthlingtonson the 14th. It really made me laugh and put me in a great mood. I haven't laughed so hard in ages and can't wait to hear about tomorrow's episode of the blue elephants! He refused to play the guitar for me though but that was ok. I gave him a massage so he would sleep better.

171

My View on the Place: After I had left I soon started to hate it. Having once felt so secure and protected there I soon started to disagree with everything the staff had taught me to believe. I still to this day do not think that bodily harm is an addiction. I know that I personally will not start shaking violently if I have not had my razor fix. I think that for some people with a serious addiction it can be and is helpful. However, for anyone who is a self harmer, an anorexic or has a mental disorder it is not the place. The staff are not trained for this, nor are they qualified to take on those patients.

How It Affected Me: It confused me. I left knowing no more about myself than I did when I went in. I was angry with the staff but also grateful to them. Some had made lasting memories in my mind and I still laugh at the thought of what they got up to. I did leave with more confidence as well as a few good friends who I am still in contact with today. That is about the only good thing that came out of my experience. Harry, Sam, Brent and Alice died of overdoses or suicide within a few months of leaving the London Half way house. They are greatly missed.

WHO?

Who decides normality?
Who knows what reality is?
Who defines sanity?
Who can give me clarity?

RESEMBLANCE

The silent storm of emotions inside,
Angry and tense,
Tears fall from my eyes,
When I hear your footsteps,
Your voice glides among the wind,
My fear starts to grow,
I feel you all around me,
Cold like winter snow,

172

I try to think why this chilled scene,
Should bring back such remembrance,
And why every man I see,
Screams out your resemblance,
Every violent yell grabs my attention,
Memories of feeling deserving,
For everything you did to me,
I'm scared of every corner I'm turning,
Because each dark shadow,
Contains your very portrait.

HOW?

How can I smile at the world,
If it doesn't smile at me?

How can I speak,
When I don't have a voice?

How can I feel so numb,
When I slice just to bleed?

How can I get better,
When I don't have a choice?

How can I ask for help,
When I don't know how?

How can I release my pain,
When I can never cry?

How can I think of the future,
When I can't even think of now?

How can I breathe,
When all I want is to die?

CHAPTER TEN

London-3 Half-Way House

November-January
18 years old

Arrival: It was dark outside. I was in an ally way with mews houses lining the thin road. I was showed to a small house that had bedrooms and told that that was where I would sleep. My room had two beds and a closet. I was not used to the traffic that I heard outside or the lingering stuffy air that cocooned the city. It was so loud compared to Kent. It felt as if I had been taken from a womb and was now in the real world. I didn't have the safety of the bubble wrapped house in the country.

First Impression: It was like a mini replica of the manor house. I was shown around by a girl I knew from Kent. She who had once looked so healthy in leaving now had bags under her eyes and greasy hair. A fake smile was worn well on her face, but she was not the girl I had once known. I knew she was using again. I started doubting my own recovery. If she had been so strong and was now back with her addiction, I would be worse as I was already weakening.

BODY ARMOUR

Scar tissue does not have wrinkles, or hair. It is numb and has no feeling. On an old deep scar, you can prick it with a needle and not feel it. The cells are dead. I used to hurt the outside to hurt the thing on the inside. Maybe now I hurt the outside to protect the thing on the inside. It is like a piece of body armour.

Sometimes I wish it covered my entire body instead of select patches. I'm not mad enough to set myself alight, or take a bath in acid but perhaps I should make a diary date, to remind myself in three years. I just might be mad enough then.

The Professionals: The same doctor from the country and his son ran this place. I didn't see him everyday though but there was a group on Fridays. I was relieved when I found this out because I had often found his groups so draining.

The Regular Staff: The staff at the secondary centre ere the same as in the country. All of them were recovering addicts; all of them thought that the doctor was king. They didn't however seem as clued up as the last staff members and I soon found ways of manipulating them.

The Other Patients: They were not as friendly. They had already formed groups of friends so mingling was quite hard. I didn't see many of them after five as most of them went home rather than staying in the rooms. A lot of the patients didn't have as serious problems as the ones in the country did. Most of them had not even been to the country house but went straight into this place instead.

Departure: I was so happy to leave. I had made plans of where and when I was going to cut. The girl who had showed me around when I arrived had left and was back on heroin. I envied her in some way. I wanted to try it as soon as I left. I was laughing at the thought that I would have entered a rehab clean and would leave a smack head to be.

REACTIONS

People are always interested in me. They study me like some animal. They cower over me inspecting any signs of my disorder as if it was contagious. If I need to go to a boring dinner I will know the outcome before going. I find normal people so predictable and repetitive.

There will be the middle aged housewives whose children have all been sent to boarding school. They ask questions but not because they are concerned about me but more of a checklist. They chit chat amongst themselves about the symptoms and compare which of their children have them. If their spawn has them they either go over the top in trying to explain their kids are perfectly normal, or demand a list of top psychiatrists. They live their lives in denial that they could have possibly reproduced or created a sick child. They munch up medication from their doctors and claim it is because of stress. Their argument is that they are prescribed which they know is acceptable among their circle of friends.

Then there are the well educated men who will use me as an example of politics and the education system, and go to extremes to prove their points. They will throw around large words that I could never remember how to say let alone understand. They pretend to know all the clinical words and phrases and will often quote a psychological study on teenagers they read in a newspaper. They think any allegations that some parents are to be held responsible for their defected child are wrong and will defend them with their life. They talk to me in a patronising voice and never listen to my opinions because of whom I am.

There will be the rebellious sons who know I will displease their parents, and so would love to date me purely for that reason. Begging me if I could just meet their family suggesting I shouldn't bother with long sleeves. They try and relate to my experiences and claim they are so depressed for some petty reason. They admire me, think my disorder is cool and state that suicide is in this season.

There will be the junkies who believe they can relate to me because I hate life. They will use their time talking to me about which doctors are easy to get methadone from and which psychiatrists they have done coke with. They will carefully go through which doctors I have seen and demand any gossip about them. If I have none they will fill me in on which ones are easy to manipulate, which ones are good and which ones they reckon they can fuck. They will compare their track marks with my scars and ask if needle fetishes are the same with my love for sharp blades. They will give me numbers of good pimps and dramatically tell a story of their experience with hallucinations. After all that they are either amazed that I am not a smack head, or try to pressure me to shoot up with them.

Wherever I go or whoever I speak to people want to know. They need to know that they are not like me that they can never turn into someone like me and if they do, where they should go. I stopped telling people about myself a while ago. When I realised how much shit I get.

My View on the Place: Like zombies patients would go round acting just like the doctor. Many idolised him for saving them from their lives. It could be helpful if you have an addiction but again it was not a place to be if you are a bit crazy like me.

How It Affected Me: I left worse off than when I went in. I had started cutting before I left and not many patients seemed bothered by it at all. I started to not bother hiding my cuts as I had done for so many years. My thoughts were mixed up. I had gone there to try and get some clarity as to whom I was and why I did the things I did. I feel that I got none of these things. To every question I asked, addict was the answer. I soon was so mixed up and fragile that I had no sense of who I was, am or used to be. I wanted to turn to drugs. I was going to shoot smack up into my veins, just for the hell of it. I did not care anymore. If I didn't know who I was then why should it matter if I existed? I felt isolated, incurable and I saw no sense in me living. I felt guilty that my parents had wasted more time and money on me, when I was not getting better. I started hanging with junkies and people who slept on the street. I wanted to sell my body and I befriended local prostitutes that I knew. I had finally an understanding of what rock bottom really was. Hope to me was now nothing more than a word in a dictionary.

THINK OF ME

Think of me,
When you don't want to live,
Think of me,
When you have nothing left to give.
Think of me,
When you're feeling down,
Think of me,
When you just want to drown.
Think of me,
When you're feeling sad,
Think of me,
When you think you are bad.
Think of me,
When you cut across your skin,
Think of me,
When you feel full of sin.
Think of me,
When you grab the knife,
Think of me,
When you want to end your life.
Think of me,
When you cry yourself to sleep,
Think of me,
When you cut too deep.
Think of me,
When the blood starts to flow,
Think of me,
When you just want to go.
Think of me,
When know one else will care,
Think of me,
When nobody's there.
Think of me,
When you want to die,
Think of me,
It might change your mind.

COMING AND GOING

Standing here nothing going my way,
Feeling black on a perfect day,
Stuffed with emotions with nothing to say,
With my flesh razors like to play.
I need help but have no one to ask,
I open up and then I run,
Desperately wanting to throw away my mask,
Laughing at my disorder but it's not fun.
Wondering why I'm stuck in this place,
Covering up the bruises on my face,
My mind blank an empty space,
Perhaps I really am a nut case.

ESTHER

Her life; a story untold
Faded tracks on her arms
A sweet innocent smile
That raises the alarm.
Beyond the frayed edges
Is a girl that once was gone
Now a mature woman
Whose happiness is a song.
Her anger floats away
And her daughter shows a smile
All that once was lost
Returns for a while.
Her laughter is infectious
Eternal memories deranged
The bend in the path we walked
Forever goes unchanged.

NEW HORIZONS

I am suffocating.
A cloud is surrounding me
Heavy as a blanket and thick.
It is not grey but yellow.
Rays of light reach out to me

179

I try and run in fear.
I am trapped.
Enclosed in a cave
Holding me within its walls.
Like a prisoner I can't escape.
It is not empty but full
Of happiness and joy.
I am paralysed.
An overwhelming feeling inside me
Something new and uncomfortable.
A difference I can't get used to.
I want back my darkness
Me shadows that I hide in.
I am lost.
My future has been written
It does not end in suicide.
Threatening words of love.
Recovery grasping me
My outlook is unfortunately hopeful.
I am scared.
Wrapped up in cotton wool.
Peace and calm clinging to me.
Making my skin itch with joy.
Not in control, nor depressed
I have to face the facts
I am actually getting better.

THE PROMISED BUBBLE

I have a picture of us all,
We who have lived within a bubble,
Ruining our pathetic lives,
Always getting into trouble.
Our lives collided into each others,
But some smiles are now faded,
In the photo we were laughing and having fun,
Now a few of those lives have been wasted.
Yes our bodies needed rest,
And our souls wanted the healing,
Thrown in at the deep end,
So forced into feeling.

What happened after that summer was gone,
After we had all reawakened,
We went into our new world so prepared,
For some we were mistaken.
Real or fake stories of life ever after,
How our recovery would win,
We fooled our minds into believing the tale,
Forgetting the strength of our sin.
Connected by the fact we were different,
Together our insanity had stopped,
But when alone in real life, we soon realised,
The bubble, our safety had popped.

CHAPTER ELEVEN:

OUT OF TREATMENT

Living on your own in a new place, in a new home, in a new city is hard. If you're my age it is very hard. If you have just spent two years in a hospital, it is almost impossible.

I was used to a nurse waking me up, feeding me my meals, giving me medication and a nurse watching me have a shower. I was used to going to sleep to a riot. My mornings usually involved watching a restraint in progress. I was used to walking round without shoes. Twice a day I had to have a body search.

I wasn't used to music, the sunlight, telephone calls, shopping, cleaning and bills. Well I'm still not good at bills, but I am improving. I was not used to walking my dog, cleaning up after my dog-on several occasions-or having this living drooling thing rely on me completely.

At first it was weird, well it still is sometimes, not being in there. Not being in that dark place. For such a long time my nights were too quiet. I was used to shouting and some one screaming for hours, I was used to flash lights being shone at me every fifteen minutes. I was used to heavy sedatives to put me to sleep. I was not used to the silence, that deadly silence that crept into my flat and covered me. It would not end. It went on, and on. I would lie there in that silence, that deadly silence and pray to hear a scream. I would want to hear someone crying, but I never did.

I had to learn to leave the television on. It was on every minute, every hour for about four months. So were all the lights, and the radio. My poor bank account. I have only now just managed to have silence during the day. In fact dare I say it, I almost like it. At night however the radio is on. I have not managed to handle silent nights yet, but give me a break I'm still adjusting. Yes even though it's been over a year since I left hospital.

As for bills - don't go there. Ask me in maybe three or four years, I just might be ready to control them then. I think. I'm not making any promises.

Shopping: again, not being controlled as well as it should but hey, I'm only twenty, so I will justify it as much I as want to thank you.

Cleaning my own flat is going ok now, when I have the energy. I am sleeping a lot better even though I am off my beloved sedatives. My dog is being taken care of very well. Spoilt rotten if I am to be honest, but he isn't complaining.

I am getting alot better at organising myself, my time, and my life - not yet. I keep my appointments – well most of them and I am starting to feel more and more happy in the real world. That place I thought I could never live in. Well I have and I am. Yippee, for now at least.

BIG SISTER AND LITTLE SISTER

There was a time where you were the little sister and I was the big sister. There was a time when I wasn't like I am now. There was a time where you believed in me because I was your big sister. You listened to me, and trusted me and were proud of me because I was your big sister.

When mum and dad would yell at me, you would start to cry for me because I was your big sister. When I was in trouble you would say it wasn't my fault because I was your big sister. When I was scared at night I would run into your room and you would let me lie there beside you because I was your big sister. I knew all the secrets about your class mates because I was your big sister and when you had hurt yourself you would call out for me because I was your big sister. When you had your first crush you told me because I was your big sister. When I had no friends you would let me play with yours because I was your big sister.

When I was smoking behind our old Wendy house I told you to take a drag and you did because I was your big sister. When Hattie and I got drunk at the pub you kept an eye on me because I was your big sister. When I started self harming you kept it a secret because I was your big sistes and when I went into hospitals you sent me little letters because I was your sister. You would call me and tell me you loved me because I was your big sister.

When I came out it wasn't the same I was no longer your big sister. When things happened in your life I was the last one to find out because I was no longer your big sister. I never knew who your boyfriend was because I was no longer your big sister and you never told me your dreams anymore because I was no longer your big sister. We never cuddled and talked anymore because I was no longer your big sister and the secrets you told your friends you didn't tell me because I was no longer your big sister. You resented me and you were angry with me because I was no longer your big sister. There was no time for me; I was too difficult because I was no longer your sister.

So I wondered and was confused because I missed my own little sister. I wanted and needed so desperately my own little sister. I couldn't find her anymore my own little sister. She had disappeared, my own little sister. I had a memory long ago of my own little sister. I loved beyond any reasonable understanding my own little sister. I wished for the closeness I had once had with my own little sister. I wanted her to return to me because she was my very own special little sister.

GETTING BETTER

Getting better is a funny thing. You don't notice it at first. It creeps up on you slowly. It's only when you

184

realise all the scars on your arms have healed and there are no new ones. Or when a doctor asks you when the last time you heard your voices was, and you have to try and remember. That's when your heart starts pounding and you shake because you know you are doing well, and are getting better.

I didn't like it at first. It was new to me and uncomfortable. It was also strange and scary. It meant recovery. Recovery meant friends, a job, no medication, and no excuse to not do normal things. Most of all it meant to be like everyone else. Recovery to me meant normal. It didn't mean happiness, but instead boring, average and worst of all acceptance.

I had craved all those things before. But now these normal things were lined up for me waiting for me to try them and I didn't like it. Usually when I find my self getting better and I notice my arms are scab and stitch free, I go on a massive cutting bender. Just to prove to my self I am still ill. Self harm then turns into something different. No longer do I need it, but instead I use it to stay the same.

When you cut just to stay ill it is horrible. It hurts so badly. It takes so much effort to make even the smallest incision. You feel dizzy and sick sometimes. When you cut because you really need it; you don't feel the pain as much. Your inner pain is so big and you desperately need to cut that it isn't the same.

Recovery I thought was evil. It was as if it grabbed me by the throat and pulled me into its happiness. I wanted the borderline to come and grasp me back into the darkness.

It did. It still does just not as often. It took me a while to realise that recovery did not mean normal. I would always be me no matter what. It meant that I would have relief from some tiring behaviours. It also meant that I would never be like every one else. I would be fine then go back to my old ways, then do better etc...

185

After a long time I started liking it. My voices were decreasing a lot and my depression was not as bad. I realised it wasn't as much fun as I thought to stay sick.

I still cut sometimes and when I am very stressed out I will have my voices but they are not half as bad as they used to be. My relationships with men got better and I stopped attacking them with my illness. Most importantly of all I stopped wanting to die and started wanting to live instead.

HOME

After you have had to deal with all your issues inside of a treatment centre or nut house, and have been cared for and helped, they spit you out. They protect you from the cruel world, they shelter and protect you, and then they pack your bags and show you to the door.

Nothing prepares you. All your coping strategies, that have been drilled into your memory get lost and forgotten when you see that first look. The look in people's eyes when they know where you have been. The one that says, "I know who you are!" sometimes it is in the form of a nod, but instead as a little smirk or side comment.

You leave so confident. So sure of who you are and that you can live a normal life, and then you realise that that is not the case. That there is no possibility of living in a normal world with normal people who try and forget people like us exist.

After realising that once you are out there, no one understands you, you start to want to go back. Needing protection you discover how easy it was being locked up. The thought of being away from the sane world once scared you but now you are desperate for it.

Inside is a place where you are understood. A place where your weird thoughts and behaviours are not laughed at usually, and where a little pill can help you sort out your feelings and problems.

It can also be hell, a place where you wouldn't wish your worst enemy to be in. Where for years later you will still have nightmares of what staff members and other patients did to you. However even with the worst experiences you can possibly have in a psychiatric unit, there is still something that it can provide you. It's something that the normal world cannot.

No matter how hard you try and deny it, and wonder confusingly how it is possible, you have to accept that you miss it and that it is safe. It's certainly not in some ways. It cannot protect you as well as it should from the insane. It cannot always stop a riot from happening or a patient killing themselves. They can't always prevent a patient trying to hurt you, a staff member trying to rape you and often fail at protecting you from yourself.

They do however protect you from something worse. A thing that scares every patient because it is the one and only thing we cannot understand, sanity. Some patients will experience it, others never will, but it is always dreaded. As long as we are kept away from the happy people with perfect lives, and the overly cheerful weather girls who make us physically sick, we will be o.k.

It helps us feel normal when we are not. It lets us know we are understood and that we are not alone. It creates a place, and perhaps the only place where we can fit in. It's where we feel whole.

In that place we know that scars are not stared at, hallucinations are not thought badly of, where starving yourself is not new or weird, and that rape almost everyone can relate to.

It is when you leave, you realise these few things do not exist outside and that people like us are huddled into a group with a label. We are not normal anymore

187

and certainly not as accepted by those who do not understand. It is then that you realise that a psychiatric unit, hospital, treatment centre or nut house is your sanity. It is your home.

MY OWN PACE

My own pace is something that I have always done, and am doing now. I refuse to let people tell me how to live my life when they don't realise that up till now I have not had one. I will not listen to my father when he tells me to start doing some courses, or try and do my A levels. I will not take advice from therapists who claim that to get a few degrees, to pass a few exams, to study in a university with permanently happy students will give me a chance in life. I do not pretend anymore, I have spent years lying to concerned faces, telling them I am happy. I will not go back to that.

I will not walk the halls with note books and pens, a painted smile on my face and long sleeves to cover my history. Joining in with people my own age who have no clue of what life, unhappiness is all about. I will not let my goal in life be to ask some guy in my class to go out with me. I will not let my happiness rest on what I will wear at a club on Saturday night. I will not experience life by getting drunk and throwing up on my best mate. Or popping a little white pill so that I can hug everyone - it would be fun, but no.

I do not need that to know who I am. I know who I am and who I always will be. I know more about my disorder than most therapists and psychologists that try and treat me. I know what it is like to lose everything; my family, my friends, my dignity and my sanity. I know true desperation to end a life. I know the tempting of the razors edge. I know forced sex, medications, voices, depression. I do not know normality but no one does, even if they claim so.

The only important thing about life, to me is to survive it. I judge a day on whether I have used my razor or not. I will do whatever it is that makes me happy. My life as a patient, as a Borderline is too short.

Wow, I really am in a black mood today. Maybe it is just because it is 2:00am - well I did say that I needed to work on my sleep patterns - see I do not think I am perfect.

My own pace is what some might call slow. Then again those that call it slow live in the real world, the city, the fast lane. I take my time. I am fine with that. As long as I am organized, getting things done and enjoying life then I am happy. As long as I am not getting so tired I am depressed, or needing to cut, I am happy - as long as my psychiatrist is happy, I am happy.

LOVE IS ALL THE SMALL THINGS

It's all the small things that you do
When no one is around and it's just me and you.
 It's all the little secrets that we share
And the way a single kiss can show me that you care.

It's the words you whisper, softly in my ear
Your protective arms around me driving out my fear.
It's how we have arguments but look back at them and smile
When you hold me and the world stops for a while.

It's the way you don't realise that there is food on your cheek
And how you murmur whenever you are asleep.
It's the little look you give me to tell me something's wrong
When I am depressed you help me to carry on.

It's when you sing in the shower, you don't think I can hear
How even though I can't see you, I know when you are near.
It's the way when the phone rings; I know that it is you
And when you tell me you believe in all that I do.

It's how you hold me tightly when you don't want me to
go
How I don't need to tell you things, because you
already seem to know.
It's how we'll both say the same thing at the same time
All these things let me know, I love you and you are
mine.

NEW AWAKENING

A day I'd guessed would never come
The thought of it made me quite numb
I had never known that this could happen
A christening was not part of the pattern.
The church was towering overhead
I had been there before to bury the dead
Last time the sky was dark and grey
But now blue heaven and a sunny day.
It made me smile to see her so
Before dressed in black and had wanted to go
Now I floated in a sea of smiles
Instead of white lilies, presents in piles.
To know that when one soul will leave
Another arrives, bundled to please
To think that life keeps on going
That my soul keeps on growing.

MARC'S NO-MAN'S LAND

The angry eyes, still haunting
His body is made of sand,
Now a drifting shadow
That lurks in no-mans land.
He has gone to join the army
Of his peers that all are damned.
Shifting in amongst them
A bottle in his hand.
Lack of understanding
Within his fragile mind,
The leaves have all fallen

190

But they land on ground that is kind.
Below the cherry blossoms
That bloom with such pride,
A tainted figure lingers
In darkness he will hide.
Memories half forgotten
With every poisonous sip,
When walking life's crooked path
Make sure not to trip.

UNLOCK THE DOOR

Enter through the ebony coloured door,
Into the deepest realms of my mind,
Past the screeching wind torn trees,
And tell me what you find.

Around the blazing fires that roar,
Take the path across my crackling soul,
Climb up the jagged, sharp edged cliffs,
And tell me that I am whole.

Entwine within the darkest shadows,
Try ignore the sorrow filled scream,
Dodge the blood-thirsty beasts that howl,
And tell me what you see.

Walk confidently towards the sharpened razors,
Do not dare to hate the pain,
Let your blood feed my emotions,
And tell me that I am sane.

A DRINK OF NOTHING

He sleeps beside me, my lover,
Without knowing who I am,
He takes a sip or two,
Trying to understand.

At first his tongue would lick,

Like a child tasting a finger of wine,
But know he drinks me in whole,
Downing me though I decline.

In large long gulps he forces,
Who I am down his gut,
Pint after pint of personality,
An intoxicating mixture of angel and slut.

His liver damaged by my memories,
Concentration distracted by my fears,
Shaking and rattling from my love,
His forehead stained with lines of tears.

Without me he is helpless,
A wrecked shell without a soul,
But with me, he is dying,
In his heart I've carved a hole.

He drinks, and swallows nothing,
Refusing to believe he is wrong,
He can't get drunk on my sanity,
My sanity is long gone.

MY TAINTED ANGEL

Hiding in the corner,
With his wings tucked in,
Alone in a world full of hatred,
There is no one to soothe him.
His eyes look inoffensive,
Not willing to show his fear,
Behind hazel-green there is despondency,
In torment and tears.
His childhood has been stolen,
Feelings forever locked away,
Lost in a world so darkened,
Like this I don't want him to stay.
No one to comfort him,
Or soothe away the pain,
His wings are withered,

192

Constantly caught in the rain.
Fallen from heaven,
A boy trying to be a man,
Hands clenched into fists,
Trying to understand.
He once was innocent,
Now tears in his eyes,
He grew up too fast,
His life he does despise.
I will not give up hope,
Though he is no longer divine,
Needing, but fearing love,
This sweet soul is mine.
Through darkness I will lead him,
In shadows part of him always will dwell,
But I believe in him,
My love, my tainted angel.

TIMES ARE CHANGING

Blue moon
Moonbeam
That's how I dreamt of you
A dream so serene.
Star light
In the night
That's when my wish came true
For you.

Together
Apart
But you have lived in my heart
Now I'm blue
Waiting for love anew.

Sometimes
And never
You will be with me
And leave forever.

I will see
Winter will always come
To sing to me.

In a cage I'm free
Touching sands
Walking with the sea
In hands.
I believe
My future
Written with sand
Will be.
Our life
Death and us
Highway makes a 'U' turn.

A FINAL WISH

Marc Why do you have to go
Into that dark pit of hatred?
Catching feelings spinning
Round the room once tasted.
Only to be analysed
Pointed at and patronised
To be told what you already know
Your life is wasted.

Why do you have to be
Torn from the world that is spinning?
To realise the devil clinging
To your back is winning.
Where everyone looks the same
They think you are playing a game
To be kicked out of the group
Because the negative is ringing.

Why do you have to scream
At night to get attention?
Flying through red memories
Demanding your redemption.

194

No one knows how you feel
It's a dream it can't be real
You beg for just one soul
To grant you some appreciation.

Why have you been grabbed
Out from your safety net?
All this talking all the time
Just fills your heart with regret.
Now your tale has been sold
With promises that you'll grow old
Keep bringing up the past
When you just want to forget.

THE END

DOCUMENTARIES IN THE MEDIA

"Inside Out." Channel 4, 1995.
"Damage." Channel 5, 1997.
"East." BBC 2, 2000.
"The Secret Of Seroxat." BBC's Panorama, October 14th, 2002.

ARTICLES IN POPULAR PRESS

Favazza, A, and Conterio, K. "The Plight Of Chronic Self-Mutilators." Community Mental Health Journal, 1988.
Favazza, A, and Contario, K. "Female Habitual Self-Mutilators." Psychiatric Scandinavia, 1989. Nakhla, F, and Jackson, G. "Picking Up The Pieces." Yale University Press, 1993.
Shappell, E. "The Unkindest Cuts." Allure, August, 1995. Todd, A. "Razor's Edge." Seventeen, June, 1996.
Pedersen, S. "Girls Who Hurt (Themselves)." Sassy, June, 1996. Egan, J. "Cutting." New York Times Magazine, July 27th, 1997. Green, J. "Living on the Edge." North Star, October, 1997.
Rubin, S. "The Unkindest Cut." San Francisco Chronicle, October 11th, 1998. Strong, M. "The Bright Red Scream." Viking Press, 1998.
Pool, B. "Cutters," Learn How To Heal Their Scars. Los Angeles Times, April 6th, 2002.
"Borderline Personality." Harvard Mental Health Newsletter, 2002.
Goetz, K. "Reasons Vary, But Forms Of Self-Mutilation Date's Back Centuries." Cincinnati Enquirer, July 28th, 2002.
Goetz, K. "Cutting Through The Pain." Cincinnati Enquirer, July 28th, 2002.

BOOKS:-
(RECOMMENDED READING FOR
PROFFESIONALS, FAMILY, PATIENTS AND
ANYONE WITH A GENERAL INTREST IN SELF-
HARM AND MENTAL ILLNESS.)

The book we recommend above all others is Robinson,
L & Cox, V. Voices Beyond the Border.
Chipmunkapublishing, 2006.

Alderman, T. The Scarred Soul: Understanding and
Ending Self-Inflicted
Violence. Oakland, CA: New Harbinger, 1997.
American Psychiatric Association. Diagnostic and
Statistical manual of Mental
Disorders, 4th ed. Washington, D.C.: 1994.
Contario, K., Lader, W., and Jennifer Kingston Bloom.
Bodily Harm: The
Breakthrough Healing Program For Self-Injurers. New
York, Hyperion,
1998.
Brumberg, J. The Body Project: An Intimate History of
American Girls.
New York: Random House, 1997.
Favazza, Armando. R. Bodies Under Siege: Self-
Mutilation and Body
Modification in Culture and Psychiatry. 2nd ed.
Baltimore: Johns
Hopkins University Press, 1996.
Fox, C. and Hawton, K. Deliberate Self-Harm in
Adolescence. Jessica Kingsley
Publishers, 2004.
Friedel, R.O. Borderline Personality Disorder
Demystified. Marlowe &
Company, 2004.
Gunderson, J.G. Borderline Personality Disorder: A
Clinical Guide. American
Publishing Inc, 2001.
Kaplan, L, J. Female Perversions. New York:
Doubleday, 1991.

Kaysen, S. Girl Interrupted. Virago Press Ltd, Little, Brown and Company,
London, 2000.

Kernberg, O. F. Severe Personality Disorders: Psychotherapeutic Strategies.
New Haven: Yale University Press, 1986.
Kettlewell, C. Skin Game: A Memoir. St. Martin's Griffin, 2000.
Kroll, J. The Challenge of the Borderline Patient: Competency in Diagnosis and
Treatment. New York: W. W. Norton, 1998.
Kreisman, J. and Stratus, H. I Hate You--Don't Leave Me. Los Angeles:
The Body Press, 1989.
Kriesman, J. and Straus, H. Sometimes I Act Crazy: Living with Borderline
Personality Disorder. John Wiley & Sons Inc, 2004.
Latza, K., Contario, K. and Lader, W. Understanding and Treating the
Self-Injurious Patient: An Audiotape for Professionals (110 minutes),
1996. Published by SAFE Alternatives.
Leatham, V. Bloodletting: A True Story of Secrets, Self-Harm and Survival.
Allison & Busby, 2005.
Levenkron, S. Cutting: Understanding and Overcoming Self-Mutilation.
W.W.Norton & Co Ltd, New York, 1999.
Mason, P.T. and Kreger, R. Stop Walking on Eggshells: Coping When Someone
You Care About Has Borderline Personality Disorder. New Harbinger
Publications, 1998.
McCormick, P. Cut. CollinsFlamingo, 2002.
Menninger, Karl. Man Against Himself. New York: Harcourt Brace, 1938.
Miller, D. Women who Hurt Themselves: A Book of Hope and Understanding.
New York: Basic Books, 1994.
Moskovitz, R.A, Lost in the Mirror: An Inside Look at Borderline Personality

Disorder. Taylor Trade Publishing, 2001.

Pegler, J. A Can of Madness. Chipmunkapublishing, 2004.

Pipher, M. Reviving Ophelia: Saving the Selves of Adolescent Girls. New
York: Ballantine, 1994.

Plath, S. The Bell Jar. Faber and Faber, 2001.

Reiland, R. Get Me Out of Here. My Recovery from Borderline Personality
Disorder. Hazeldon Information & Educational Services, 2004.

Santoro, J. and Cohen, R. The Angry Heart: Overcoming Borderline Personality
Disorder and Addictive Disorders. New Harbinger Publications, 1997.

Shengold, L. Soul Murder: The Effects of Childhood Abuse and
Deprivation. New York: Ballantine, 1989.

Schiller, L. and Bennet, A. The Quiet Room: Journey out of the Torment of
Madness. Little, Brown and Company, 1996.

Smith, C. Cutting It Out: A Journey Through Psychotherapy and Self-Harm.
Jessica Kingsley Publishers, 2005.

Strong, M. A Bright Red Scream: Self-Mutilation and the Language of
Pain. Virago Press, 2000.

Sutton, J. Healing the Hurt Within. How To Books, 2005.

Turner, U.J. Secret Scars: Uncovering and Understanding the Addiction of Self-
injury. Hazeldon Information & Educational Services, 2002.

Turp, M. Hidden Self-Harm: Narratives from Psychotherapy. Jessica Kingsley
Publishers, 2002.

van der Kolk, B.A. Psychological Trauma. Washington, D.C.: American
Psychiatric Press, 1987.

Villgran, N.E. New Hope for People with Borderline Personality Disorder.
Crown Publications, 2002.

Walker, A. and Gunderson, J.G. The Courtship Dance of the Borderline.
iuniverse.Com, 2001.
Walsh, B. W. and Rosen, P. M. Self-Mutilation: Theory, Research, and
Treatment. New York: Plenum, 1987.
Wirth-Cauchen, J. Women and Borderline Personality Disorder: Symptoms and
Stories. Rutgers University Press, 2001.

www.ingramcontent.com/pod-product-compliance
Lightning Source LLC
Chambersburg PA
CBHW031159270326
41931CB00006B/330